DIY AROMATHERAPY

Over 130 Affordable Essential Oil Blends
for Health, Beauty, and Home

FOREWORD BY LEA HARRIS
Certified Clinical Aromatherapist

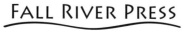

FALL RIVER PRESS

New York

FALL RIVER PRESS

New York

An Imprint of Sterling Publishing Co., Inc.
1166 Avenue of the Americas
New York, NY 10036

ISBN 978-1-4351-6418-5

For information about custom editions, special sales, and premium and corporate purchases,
please contact Sterling Special Sales at 800-805-5489 or specialsales@sterlingpublishing.com.

Manufactured in China

2 4 6 8 10 9 7 5 3 1

www.sterlingpublishing.com

CONTENTS

Foreword by Lea Harris 7

Introduction 9

I
AROMATHERAPY 101

CHAPTER 1
AROMATHERAPY BASICS
13

CHAPTER 2
SHOPPING FOR AROMATHERAPY PROJECTS
29

CHAPTER 3
YOUR FIRST AROMATHERAPY BLENDS
39

II
OILS AND REMEDIES FOR HEALTH, BEAUTY & HOME

CHAPTER 4
35 OILS TO KNOW AND USE
49

CHAPTER 5
REMEDIES FOR HEALTH & HEALING
87

CHAPTER 6
REMEDIES FOR COSMETIC CARE
161

CHAPTER 7
REMEDIES FOR THE HOME
193

CHAPTER 8
PERFUME RECIPES
221

Measurement Conversions 231

Glossary 232

Quick Reference Guide to Aromas and Oils 234

Resources 235

References 241

Index of Essential Oils 243

Index 245

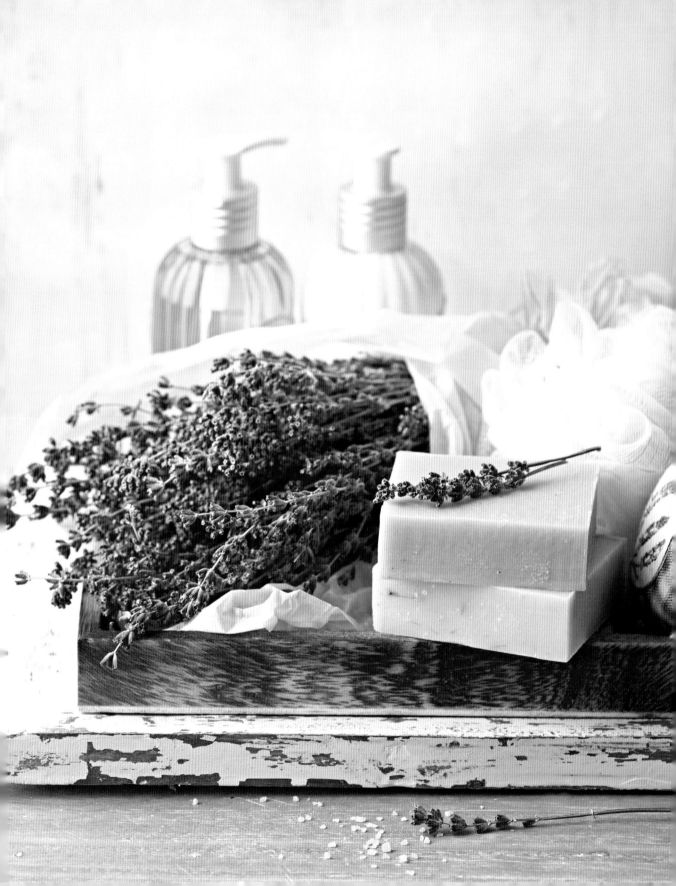

FOREWORD

Aromatherapy is a growing industry, and more and more people are becoming interested in learning about and using essential oils. As you may already know, essential oils are very concentrated plant substances. It is our job to learn what we can about them and use them in our homes and on our bodies with great care. One drop of an essential oil might come from thousands of pounds of flower petals, and it might take just one diluted drop to soothe your bug bite.

As a Certified Clinical Aromatherapist and aromatherapy blogger, I receive questions all the time from those who follow my blog. Most often, I hear from readers when they stumble across recipes in their online travels and wonder if they're safe. I guess word has traveled that I am a bit of a safety geek. When you don't have a trusted, go-to resource, it can be overwhelming to figure out where to start.

Odds are that you know just a little bit about essential oils and you're eager to dive right in. That's how I was when I first found out about EOs and all that they could offer. But you need to be careful which resources you

> There are so many essential oils, and they can be useful for a variety of issues. Knowing when and how to use them is key to aromatherapy success.

choose. I bought several books geared to beginners when I started my aromatherapy journey. But after I received aromatherapy training, I realized they were full of unsafe information. I haven't touched them since. By purchasing and using this book, you'll avoid making the same mistake I did.

It's natural to assume that because essential oils originate from plant sources they are without risk, but this is not always the case. There are safety issues to consider when you use them. If you have children in your home, there are essential oils you'll want to avoid using around them. Pregnant women need to use caution, as there are some essential oils known to cause harm to a growing baby when misused. Some essential oils can elicit bad reactions if applied topically and the skin is exposed to the sun. All essential oils should be diluted before topical use, some require extra dilution, and it goes without saying that essential oils should never be used internally without guidance from a professional aromatherapist who has received training in aromatic medicine.

DIY Aromatherapy is a great place to start experimenting safely and affordably with essential oils. This book tells you about the history of aromatherapy, and then goes on to explain how essential oils are made, the ways in which they work, how to choose and use them, which supplies are useful, how to make your own blends at home . . . and that is just what you'll find in the first part! In the second part of the book, you'll get to read profiles of dozens of essential oils to help you familiarize yourself with their

properties, uses, precautions—and even their scents and costs. Following the profiles is what you're really waiting for, and it's my favorite section, too. There you'll find the recipes. Included are recipes for health and wellness, cosmetic applications, perfume blends, and recipes for use in the home.

There are so many essential oils, and they can be useful for a variety of issues. Knowing when and how to use them is key to aromatherapy success. *DIY Aromatherapy* will be an indispensable guide on your fragrant journey.

Lea Harris
Certified Clinical Aromatherapist
UsingEOsSafely.com

INTRODUCTION

For centuries, people have used the potent essences of plants to heal, restore, and protect themselves from illness and injuries, and to treat day-to-day maladies. Herbal medicine has endured for good reason: It works. You might not know it, but herbs are very likely already an essential part of your health, beauty, and home-care routines. Check the ingredient list of your facial cleansers, creams, shampoos, conditioners, deodorant, and even cough drops. Herbal extracts, including fragrant essential oils, make their way into many of these products because they are powerful and effective remedies for many everyday issues.

Essential oils trigger our bodies to function efficiently, strengthen our immunity, and fight disease. When blended in the right combinations at proper dilutions, they not only scent our homes in the most pleasant ways, they can alleviate all sorts of common health concerns—from acne, dry skin, and brittle

Herbal medicine has endured for good reason: It works.

hair to fatigue, mild depression, and stress. In this book, you'll learn about the most versatile (not to mention affordable) essential oils—including why and how they work—and have at your fingertips a collection of remedies and recipes that will empower you to create your own natural healing preparations. And you'll learn that herbal medicine doesn't have to be an all-or-nothing endeavor. Your herbal remedies can be used to complement whatever you're already doing, perhaps lessening your need for commercial products, or making those products more effective.

This book begins by introducing you to the evidence-based benefits of aromatherapy so that you have both the confidence and inspiration to jump into making your own aromatherapeutic projects. After reviewing how essential oils are produced and how they work in the body, a full review of safety precautions is offered.

Next comes the fun part: shopping for essential oils and building your home apothecary. While it is certainly possible to spend a lot of money on essential oils and equipment to prepare homemade blends, creating a budget just for essential oils is not necessary. Indeed, one of the great benefits of essential oils is how cost-effective they are, both for individual and family use. Here, you'll learn about how to buy the right essential oils (and what to be wary of when shopping), which carrier oils you might need, and the bare minimum of aromatherapy equipment you should have on hand.

This book assumes that you're eager to start making your own herbal remedies but it does not take for granted that you already have a cupboard or medicine cabinet stocked full of essential oils. In fact, there's a chapter dedicated to highlighting the versatility of just five essential oils—eucalyptus, lavender, lemon, peppermint, and tea tree. With only those five on hand, you'd be able to make dozens of the blends in this book.

The heart of *DIY Aromatherapy* is made up of more than 130 remedies and recipes for health, beauty, and home concerns. Each one not only includes preparation instructions and storage recommendations, but also tells you the scent of the blend—citrus, minty, floral, and so on—as well as how much the remedy is likely to cost (using dollar signs).

By the end of the book, you'll understand the pros, cons, benefits, and suggested uses of a range of aromatherapeutic preparations. Best of all, you'll be empowered to take charge of your own health and well-being. Soon you'll be enjoying the benefits of these powerful healing herbs using safe, effective blends that you created with love and care in your own home.

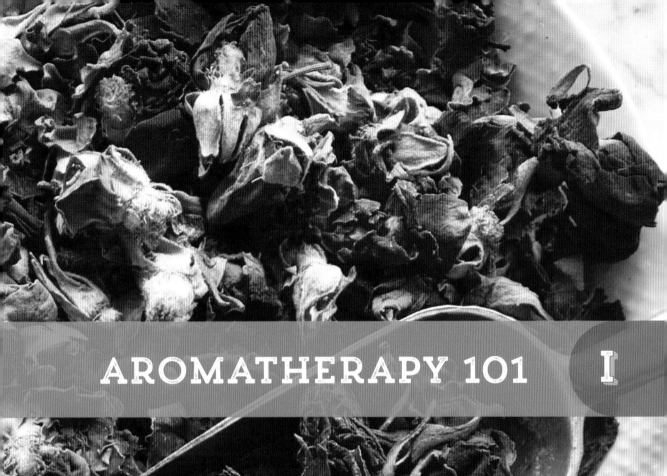

AROMATHERAPY 101   I

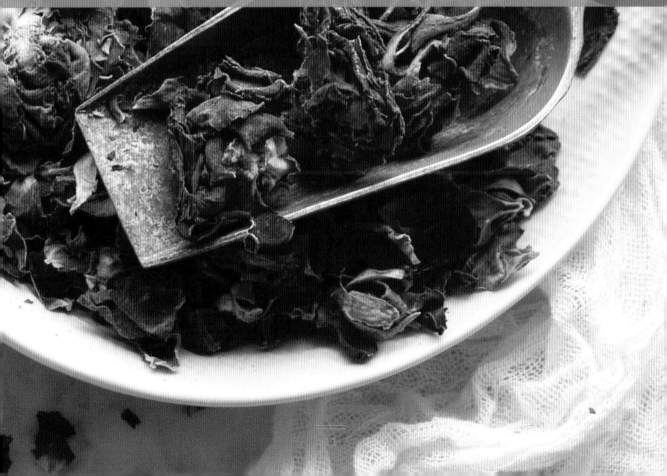

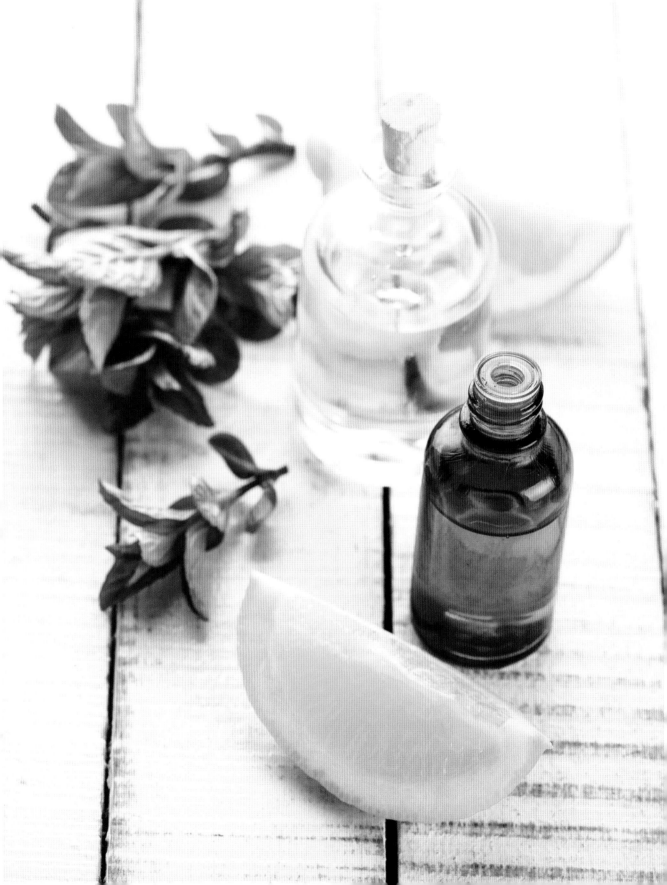

1
AROMATHERAPY BASICS

Your sense of smell is very powerful. Many species, including humans, rely partially on their sense of smell to survive. Scent has the ability to evoke memories, calm or invigorate the senses, help you wake up or fall asleep, and discern whether foods have gone bad, among many other functions. Many people think, and understandably so, given the name, that aromatherapy is purely about scents. However, aromatherapy goes far beyond the practice of simply inhaling fragrant oils.

SCENT WITH INTENT

According to the National Association for Holistic Aromatherapy (NAHA), aromatherapy can promote physical, emotional, mental, and spiritual health and balance in the body. Of primary use in aromatherapy are *essential oils*, the complex chemical substances obtained from plants. These natural substances are as prized for their powerful fragrances as they are for their healing and beauty applications. In a very true sense, aromatherapy is indeed "scent with intent," a practice in which fragrant plant compounds work to balance the body, mind, and spirit.

For many years, the concept of aromatherapy was confined to the spa industry and a range of pampering treatments such as massages, facials, or baths, in which essential oils were applied to enhance the experience. While some massage practitioners were aware of the therapeutic benefits of certain oils, such as evening primrose for easing menstrual difficulties, the use of essential oils was all about their scent.

In the 1970s, consumers began to embrace products made from natural rather than synthetic ingredients. Along with this new appreciation for unprocessed products came a new attitude toward aromatherapy. Essential oils were no longer viewed as something akin to snake oil, but as valuable, unadulterated substances that are versatile, powerful, and healing.

Essential oils have become a valued part of a holistic approach to mental, physical, and spiritual health. Rather than writing off essential oils, the international medical community is studying their medicinal effects more closely. The results are not simply encouraging; they substantiate what practitioners of herbal medicine have known for centuries. For example, a 2002 study published in the *Journal of Clinical Psychiatry* concluded that patients who suffered from severe dementia were able to reduce their agitation by 35 percent through the application of Melissa (lemon balm) essential oil. A 2012 study in *Therapeutic Advances in Psychopharmacology* analyzed how exposure to rosemary essential oil would affect cognitive performance. Researchers reported conclusively that the performance on cognitive tasks—specifically, the ability to remember to do something—of those studied "is significantly related to concentration of [rosemary essential oil] absorbed. . . with improved performance at higher concentrations." In an interview originally published 20 years ago, Dr. Marc Micozzi, then Executive Director of the College of Physicians, spoke admiringly about the growth of "alternative and complementary medicine" and his belief that a new orientation toward "self-care" and "self-cure" could be one solution to the nation's health care crisis. In other words, embracing aromatherapy empowers you to take proactive steps that may help you improve your health and well-being, potentially reducing your need for illness-related medical care.

In the recipe section of this book are dozens of essential oil blends you can craft quickly, easily, and affordably to begin working with aromatherapy at home. From the many projects and recipes in this book, you'll learn how to:

- Put together an "alternative medicine chest" filled with time-tested natural remedies.

- Blend your own fragrances, massage oils, and lotions in just a few minutes with just a few ingredients, customizing your scent to your own specifications and tastes.
- Make effective, inexpensive, and nontoxic cleaning products.
- Create your own baby and bath products free of harsh chemicals and toxic ingredients.
- Craft your own cosmetics and bath products for fun (or even profit!).
- Save money on everything from DIY dryer sheets to homemade versions of luxury eye creams.
- Create scented candles, air freshener sprays, and special essential oil blends for room diffusers to increase focus, ease tension, and promote harmony in your living and working spaces.

Let the projects on these pages inspire you.

AROMATHERAPY THEN AND NOW

The use of essential oils in medicine and cosmetics dates back to antiquity. Egyptians, Romans, and Greeks all practiced aromatherapy. The ancient Greek philosopher Theophrastus of Athens wrote a number of botanical textbooks, including one that explored how scents affect emotions, a connection that has been rediscovered by modern aromatherapists using scents such as peppermint, lavender, and various citruses to treat depression.

Aromatic resins like myrrh and cedar were used along with the oils of cinnamon and juniper in the Egyptian mummification process, and many oils and herbs were used to consecrate bodies for burial and assist the spirits in crossing to the other side.

A Persian physician perfected steam distillation around the turn of the first millennium. Rosewater, known as *golab*, is a hydrosol still extensively used in Middle Eastern cooking and perfumery. Historian Will Durant (*Civilization*) credits the Persians with being the first civilization to craft complex perfume, with a particular fondness for the scents of lily of the valley and narcissus, two flowers that are frequently mentioned in Islamic texts along with the rose, which was considered a symbol of perfection. The 14th-century Sufi poet Mahmud Shabistari's most famous work is "The Secret Rose Garden of Sa'd ud Din Mahmud," a metaphorical explanation of Sufi metaphysics.

Ancient scripture is filled with references to scented oils, ointments, and perfumes. One of the most famous is a passage in the New Testament recorded by several apostles describing the "woman of sinful nature" who bathed Jesus' feet with an expensive perfume made of "nard." Nard is a reference to "spikenard," a much-prized oil that was a component of the sacred anointing oil used in the temples.

Crusaders returned from the Middle East with exotic aromatics like black pepper, cinnamon, frankincense and myrrh (both resins), cedarwood, sandalwood, and more. Boccaccio's 14th-century masterpiece, *The Decameron*, mentions soap scented with musk and cloves and flasks of floral waters (also called "sweet waters") distilled from roses, jasmine, oranges, and lemons.

FAQ: ESSENTIAL OILS, HYDROSOLS, AND FRAGRANCE OILS: WHAT'S THE DIFFERENCE?

Essential oils, hydrosols, and fragrance oils are aromatics. Because they are derived in different ways and have different chemical properties, they are used for different purposes.

ESSENTIAL OILS are aromatic liquids derived from the various parts of a plant—from root to blossom to bark or berry. Depending on what part of the plant they come from, essential oils can have different properties and attributes. For example, cinnamon *bark* essential oil has a stronger scent than cinnamon *leaf* essential oil and is also roughly five times more expensive. Essential oils are safe for use on the body, although they are typically so powerful they need to be diluted with carrier oils (such as jojoba oil), to prevent side effects including photosensitization (a strong reaction to sunlight) or sensitization (an allergic-like reaction on the skin). While essential oils can be ingested, they are extremely potent and best used with the guidance of a trained practitioner. Use essential oils for aromatherapy and for the recipes and projects in this book.

HYDROSOLS (sometimes referred to as floral waters or flower waters) are the waters left behind from the process of distilling plant matter to extract essential oils. During the distillation process, manufacturers typically use steam or water. The resulting products are the essential oils and the water, both of which have extracted parts of the plants' essences. The essential oils contain the fat-soluble compounds while the hydrosols contain the water-soluble substances. Hydrosols have their own benefits, uses, and properties in aromatherapy, but they tend to be more fragile than essential oils, and therefore need to be kept in the refrigerator. They also tend to be less concentrated in both scent and power. Because they are weaker, hydrosols are usually gentler than essential oils. Therefore, hydrosols may work with someone in need of gentler therapies, such as infants or someone with a lot of chemical sensitivities. Chamomile hydrosol, for example, is an excellent popular remedy for teething babies.

FRAGRANCE OILS (also known as "perfume oils") are artificial scents that use synthetic chemicals to mimic the natural scents of essential oils. They are cheaper than essential oils and often used in candle and soap making as well as in cosmetic blends. Unfortunately, while fragrance oils may successfully replicate the scent of an essential oil, they do not have the other properties that make the essential oil so valuable. They are used only for fragrance and not in health care or cooking applications. Do not use fragrance oils for the projects in this book.

Roses are native to both Europe and Asia, and the flower was considered sacred to Venus and later adapted as a symbol of the Virgin Mary. Rose petals were used to scent bath water and also basins of water used for hand washing at the table. Then, as now, "attar of roses" (also known as "rose otto" or rose essential oil) was very expensive.

Essential oil–infused recipes have been found in 9th-century "leechbooks" (medical texts). They include everything from a garlic oil–enriched eye salve that may be effective against the superbug MRSA to a disinfectant solution known as "Thieves' Vinegar" or "Thieves' Oil" used to battle the Bubonic Plague in the 14th through 16th centuries. In modern times, this blend has been clinically proven to kill bacteria.

The first alcohol-based perfume ("Hungary Water") appeared in Europe in the 1300s and was allegedly created by an alchemist to restore youth and beauty to an aging queen. Hungary Water was the first known "toilet water," a formula that was used as both a fragrance and a remedy, and gave birth to whole apothecaries of simple (one ingredient) and complex toilet waters crafted from flowers, herbs, musk, and amber.

In the 18th and 19th centuries, European colonists brought their own remedies and medicinal recipes with them to the New World but soon adopted practices found among the Native Americans and First Nation people, in particular the use of birch bark tonic to reduce fever, relieve pain, and soothe inflamed flesh. In New England, the early colonists discovered that boiling the fruit of the bayberry bush yielded a fragrant wax that could be used to make candles and, unlike their candles made of tallow (animal fat), did not go rancid.

In America, the 19th century saw the rise of a new kind of toilet water. The most famous was "Florida Water" with its spicy orange-lavender scent, and "Kananga Water," which was based on ylang ylang, an essential oil prized not only for health and personal care, but also for use in rituals of home protection and spiritual cleansing. Another formula, "Hoyt's Cologne," was said to attract luck to gamblers.

Today in the Western world, aromatherapy is commonly used both at home and in professional practices. Westerners use essential oils for an array of purposes, including health, beauty, fragrance, home products, and spiritual and mental well-being. For a while, Western culture split the use of aromatic plants into two separate branches—medicinal and cosmetic. In the 21st century, however, the growing use of cosmeceuticals (cosmetics with medicinal properties) and aromapeutics (scented products with potential therapeutic benefits) once again blurred the lines. As for other cultures, such a break never occurred. Traditional Chinese and Ayurvedic medical systems, for example, still use aromatherapy in both modalities. In a modern world grown increasingly complex and toxic, the ancient tradition of aromatherapy offers not only a link to the past but also a connection to the future of spiritual, physical, and mental health.

THE SKINNY ON ESSENTIAL OILS

Getting started with essential oils in DIY projects is easy. You don't need a lot of expensive equipment. You don't need a whole pantry full of essential oils. You don't even need any special expertise. If you can shake a bottle, you can create a blend. But, like any craft, the more you know about what you're doing, the more you enjoy the results. Here are some things you need to know.

HOW ESSENTIAL OILS ARE PRODUCED

Extracting essential oils from plants is not something that can be done easily as a DIY project. It's one thing to infuse a pitcher of water with rose petals or a couple of slices of lemon and quite another to process the thousands of roses or lemons needed to produce the highly concentrated essential oil. And even if the average DIY enthusiast had access to a lavender field or a citrus orchard, the machinery and manpower required is beyond the scope of an individual.

Essential oils are extracted using one of several basic methods. The two most common are *steam distillation* and *CO2 extraction*.

STEAM DISTILLATION is the most common method for extracting essential oils. Vast quantities of aromatic plants are loaded into a machine and tightly compacted. Steam is then forced through the plant "filter," heating it up and releasing the oils as a gas. As the gas cools, it liquefies into oil and water, which is then separated. The fragrant water that's left behind by this process is a hydrosol (see page 16) and is valued in its own right.

CO_2 EXTRACTION is a process similar to steam distillation, but it uses carbon dioxide instead of water to extract the essential oil from the raw plant material. In this method, carbon dioxide is chilled to between 35 and 55 degrees Fahrenheit before being blasted through the plant material. What results is a pure essential oil that has not been even slightly altered by exposure to heat.

Other extraction methods include:

ENFLEURAGE is an ancient French technique that involves extracting the fragrance of flowers by exposing them to the sun until the essential oils leach into a fixed oil or fat. At that point, a separation process ensues that purifies the oil to make it ready for sale.

EXPRESSION (aka "cold pressing") is used mostly for extracting the essential oil from the peels of citrus fruit. In this method the fruit peels are pressed and then the oil is separated from the juice and pulp in a centrifuge. Expression is also the process used in winemaking and creating olive oil.

MACERATION sounds like a process that would involve grinding or chewing-up herbs, but it isn't. Plants are soaked in hot oil, which breaks down their cell walls to release the essential oils. The result is then filtered and bottled. The Egyptians used this method extensively in their perfume making.

SOLVENT EXTRACTION is used when flowers have too little volatile oil for other extraction methods. The essential oils are extracted with the help of chemical solvents such as methylene chloride, hexane, or benzene, and are called "absolutes." Solvent extraction is an expensive, labor-intensive process that often involves several solvent treatments. Purists do not consider absolutes to be true essential oils due to the solvent that is left behind.

The end result of these processes is a bottle of essential oil that can be used alone or in combination as part of a DIY medicine chest, cosmetic case, and home-care cabinet.

In order to create a safe and effective collection of essential oils, choose the purest and best essential oils. Price isn't always a determiner of quality. Research the various essential oil manufacturers to determine the processes they use to create the essential oils, as well as the purity of their oils, before purchasing the essential oils you want to include in your personal aromatherapy kit.

HOW ESSENTIAL OILS WORK

Essential oils have a long tradition of use in health care. However, unlike modern pharmaceuticals, essential oils have not been as extensively studied as many other substances. That's not to say, however, that there isn't scientific evidence attesting to the effectiveness of certain essential oils. There is, and research remains ongoing. Centuries of use, along with some selected clinical studies, have shown the effectiveness of aromatherapy.

Essential oils are used as a remedy in three ways:

- Inhalation
- Topical application
- Ingestion (to be used only if recommended by a qualified professional and never in home applications)

INHALATION

There are many delivery methods for inhaling essential oils, such as burning them in a candle, putting them in steam, putting them in a diffuser, or applying a few drops to a warmer that spreads the scent. According to the National Cancer Institute, the theory behind the effectiveness of inhaled essential oils is that the chemical components of the oil bind to the receptors of the brain's olfactory bulb, which affects the limbic system (your brain's emotional center). Inhalation of essential oils—especially the mints, eucalyptus, and woody and evergreen oils like cypress, spruce, and fir—is particularly efficient at loosening and clearing congestion due to a cold or flu. Some medical professionals are reluctant to whole-heartedly endorse use of essential oils as treatment options but are willing to say that the oil may contain compounds that are analgesic, anti-inflammatory, antibacterial, and antifungal.

TOPICAL APPLICATION

When used topically, essential oils must be diluted in carrier oils, which are naturally derived plant-based oils such as sweet almond oil or jojoba oil. Essential oils can also be diluted by adding a few drops to your bath. Diluting the oils helps prevent sensitization, a reaction similar to an allergy, which may occur when you use undiluted essential oils directly on your skin. Undiluted essential oils may also irritate the skin or mucous membranes. When applied topically, the oils absorb through the skin and enter the bloodstream, where they may exert various effects, such as fighting bacteria or inflammation.

Several studies have established that aromatherapy treatments—either topical or inhaled—lessened pre-surgery anxiety. Research at the University of Maryland Medical Center, particularly on the use of lavender, concluded that, "The use of herbs is a time-honored approach to strengthening the body and treating disease."

INGESTION

Unless you are working with a trained professional, you should never take essential oils internally. Some of the oils that are beneficial used topically (such as nutmeg) may be poisonous or cause irritation of the digestive tract when taken internally. Likewise, taking essential oils internally is the least effective means for getting relief from an ailment.

SYNERGY

Just as certain nutrients work in concert to boost their impact—you need vitamin C to absorb iron, and fat to absorb vitamins A, D, and E—some essential oils combine synergistically to enhance their effects on the immune system. The recipes in this book were designed to make the most of the complementary power of various essential oils.

Valerie Ann Worwood, whose book *The Complete Book of Essential Oils & Aromatherapy* is a classic in its field, recommends dozens of synergistic blends, including a blend of thyme, lemongrass, lavender, and peppermint for repelling insects; Roman chamomile, geranium, lavender, lemon, and sandalwood for sleep-inducing; and grapefruit, palmarosa, and rosemary for managing stress.

SAFETY AND ESSENTIAL OILS

Essential oils, whether applied topically or inhaled, are much safer for use than chemical-based products like household cleaners or additive-laden cosmetics. Essential oils do not linger in the body, building up to toxic levels, and when used properly, they rarely cause side effects.

SAFETY FOR EVERYONE

The essential oils, projects, and blends in this book are generally safe for everyone. However, people with individual sensitivities may need to avoid certain oils. Everyone should also observe the following safety precautions:

- To determine whether an oil or blend is safe for you, perform a patch test. Dilute one drop of the essential oil in one teaspoon of carrier oil. Then, use a cotton swab to apply a small amount of the blend to a spot on the inside of your elbow. Cover it with a bandage and check it every 30 minutes for two to three hours for a reaction, such as reddening of the skin or a rash. If you react, wash the spot immediately with soap and water, and do not use that essential oil.

- Because it is possible to develop sensitivities you haven't experienced before, if it's been a while since you've used a blend or oil, perform the patch test again.
- Avoid using the oils around the eyes, because they can cause pain and damage.
- Avoid putting oils near flames, as they are flammable.
- Always use a carrier oil for topical application because the oils may irritate skin or cause a reaction.
- Follow the ratios for blends and recipes in this book exactly.
- Give yourself a break from oils from time to time. Don't use the same oils or blends day after day, or you may build sensitivity. A good rule of thumb for frequently used oils is to use them on a five-day-on, two-day-off schedule.
- Avoid using essential oils internally unless directed by a qualified practitioner. Because oral use may be ineffective or even dangerous, none of the recipes in this book call for oral administration.
- If you've ever experienced a sensitization reaction to any essential oil (may appear as skin breakouts, hives, sensitivity, itchiness, and redness), do not use that oil again.
- Keep oils out of reach of children and pets.
- Check with your doctor if you are taking medication to ascertain there are no possible interactions or contraindications between the meds and the oils.

HOW OFTEN CAN I USE ESSENTIAL OILS?

Essential oil blends that have been properly diluted and added to beauty and bath products should be safe for daily use, or even more often. On the other hand, overusing some essential oils, particularly the "hot" ones like cinnamon and clove, can lead to skin irritation or blisters, even if properly diluted.

Frequently reapplying perfumes and other body-scent products made with essential oils can lead to a desensitized sense of smell. You've likely encountered someone before whose perfume is so heavy you can taste it in the air, or even feel like you could choke on it. And yet, if you mention that to them, they're always surprised.

How frequently you use essential oils for therapeutic uses depends on a number of factors. If you are new to using essential oils, you may only want to use them once or twice per day, building up to a frequency of three times per day as your body adapts. Using too much too soon, or using them too frequently may cause sensitization or other reactions.

Your body also metabolizes essential oils at varying rates. To allow your body to metabolize oils, you need to take some time off now and then. For example, you might want to use a blend five days on and two days off, or you may wish to use a formula for two to three weeks before taking a week or two off, or switching to a formula with similar properties using different essential oils.

- Some essential oils may increase photo-sensitivity for up to 24 hours after topical application. Use caution in the sun.
- When making your own essential oil blends, try to maintain between 1.5 percent and 3 percent of the solution of essential oils, or about three drops of essential oil per two teaspoons of carrier oil.

SAFETY FOR PEOPLE WITH ALLERGIES

True allergies are triggered by protein molecules. While essential oils do not contain proteins (they are removed during distillation), they can combine with proteins in the skin to cause an allergic reaction. However, even if you have an allergy to an essential oil used topically, you may not have one with inhalation of the scent, because there is no protein with which the plant molecules can combine. Therefore, if you have allergic reactions to certain essential oils, inhalation of the aroma may be another option.

If you have allergies, always perform a patch test. If you react to the patch test, do not try using that oil again. Avoid using essential oils that correspond with any allergies you have. For example, if you are allergic to ragweed you should avoid using chamomile essential oil on the skin.

SAFETY IN PREGNANCY

While use of essential oils throughout pregnancy is under debate, pregnant women should avoid using essential oils altogether for the first trimester. Some essential oils are abortifacient (have properties that can induce spontaneous abortion and miscarriages) or emmenagogues (have properties that stimulate menstruation). In addition to the essential oils that should be avoided by everyone, the following is an abbreviated list of the most common essential oils that **should be avoided** by pregnant or lactating women:

- Angelica
- Aniseed
- Basil
- Black Pepper
- Birch
- Calendula
- Camphor
- Cedarwood
- Cinnamon (bark or leaf)
- Clary sage
- Clove
- Cypress
- Eucalyptus
- Fennel
- Geranium
- Hyssop
- Juniper
- Mugwort
- Myrrh
- Nutmeg
- Oakmoss
- Oregano
- Parsley
- Rosemary
- Rue
- Sage
- Spanish lavender
- Spike lavender
- Tansy
- Tarragon
- Wintergreen

For a more complete list, visit the website www.learningabouteos.com. Keep in mind that there are many different kinds of lavender, and you'll be able to recognize them by their different Latin names. While Spanish or French lavender (*Lavandula stoechas*) and spike lavender (*Lavandula latifolia*) should be avoided in pregnancy, the lavender plant known as *Lavandula angustifolia* is safe.

FROM THE MASTERS

JADE SHUTES,
FOUNDER OF THE SCHOOL FOR AROMATIC STUDIES
www.theida.com

Some days, upon reflection, I stop and wonder: Do we have a relationship with the essential oils we use? And I don't mean simply that we can spout off their safety considerations, main chemical components, and the do's and don'ts. Rather, can we deeply discuss the many aspects of a given essential oil? Do we understand its nature, its abilities? Have we used it? Have we "sat" with it? Have we ventured to meet the plant from which it comes from? What are our own observations about a specific essential oil? Not from someone else's perspective, not from science, not from clinical studies or scientific papers, but from our own personal relationship with the oil.

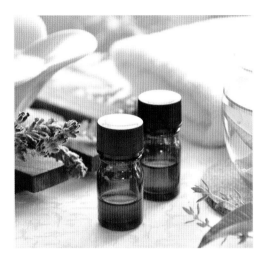

I encourage those who use essential oils to take time out and spend quality time with the essential oils, with the plants if possible, and mostly with ourselves in relationship with essential oils. Use them, smell them, read about their qualities, observe them, and deepen your relationship with them.

In the world of aromatherapy, we can be quick to use some "authority's" version of an essential oil, to become disconnected or disempowered from our own knowingness of that essential oil. Yet strength of knowledge comes not only from book knowledge but also from using, experiencing, and being in relationship with the essential oil.

Today, I encourage myself most of all to stay in relationship with essential oils by being willing to listen to their messages and allowing their "intelligence" to guide and teach me.

SAFETY FOR CHILDREN

As mentioned previously, always keep essential oils out of reach of children. If you do plan to make preparations specifically for use with children, keep these points in mind:

- You will see that many oils are described as "safe for children and babies," but they are safe only when used in specific ways. Follow recipes as written.
- With the exception of recipes formulated specifically for babies or children, assume all other recipes are formulated for adults. Adapt these recipes at **half-strength** for children 12 and under.
- Always use caution to avoid burns when administering steam inhalation treatments to children.

SAFETY FOR SENIORS

Just as children are more sensitive to essential oils than average adults, seniors—particularly, elderly and frail individuals—have heightened levels of sensitivity. Take extra care when preparing treatments intended for seniors. It's a good idea to make formulations at half-strength to prevent skin irritation or sensitization. Adjustments can be made only if there is no negative reaction after a few applications of the preparation.

ESSENTIAL OILS TO AVOID

As with anything, however, common sense applies. Some oils are so toxic they have been banned by the FDA and should not be used by anyone, in any way, under any circumstance.

Some of these include:

- Almond (bitter)
- Boldo
- Cade
- Calamus
- Camphor (Brown)
- Cassia
- Fig Leaf
- Horseradish
- Mustard
- Pennyroyal
- Sassafras
- Savin
- Snakeroot
- Tea Tree (black)
- Thuja
- Wormwood

Surprised to see tea tree essential oil on this list? Black tea tree is different from the more common tea tree that is safe for use in pregnancy. When in doubt, check the Latin name. Black tea tree is known as *Melaleuca bracteata*. The common and safe tea tree bears the Latin name *Melaleuca alternifolia*.

BLENDING OILS

To blend essential oils into a combination that's not only effective but also sensorially pleasing, you'll need to take into account both fragrance notes and aromas. Notes occur as a scent breaks down, and are layered in three parts. Top notes dominate a fragrance when you first apply it and tend to be citrusy or herbal. Middle notes arise after a few minutes and tend to be softer and more floral, such as rose. Base notes appear after about 30 minutes and may be deeper or darker, such as musk. Balanced fragrances contain an artful combination of top, middle, and base notes.

Essential oil aromas fall into broad categories. While examples are listed on page 26, this book takes out the guesswork by listing the aroma category into which each essential oil falls.

FAQ: WHICH AROMAS BLEND BEST?

When making simple blends, you don't need to worry too much about breaking down aromas, but when you're combining oils for a more complex scent, or even for a perfume, you'll want to start thinking about "notes" and how they affect the composition of the scent. A perfume's scent is like a story—it has a beginning (the "opening" or "top notes"), a middle (sometimes called the "heart notes"), and an end (the "base notes" or "the finish"). Some are longer lasting than others so a perfume can actually change its olfactory character the longer it is on your skin.

While trying out new blends is part of the fun of DIY aromatherapy, there are some guidelines you can follow so you don't waste your essential oils by making a blend that creates an unpleasant fragrance.

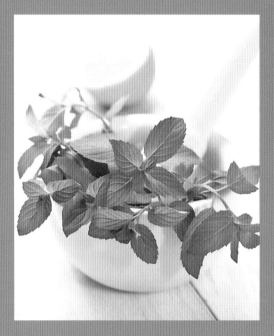

- In general, combine like with like. You can blend florals and florals, citrus and citrus, woody and woody, and so forth.

- Citrus essential oils are incredibly versatile and combine well with almost any other kind of aroma.

- Woody aromas (cedarwood, pine, spruce) also blend well across the aroma spectrum.

- Florals work with citrus, woody, and spicy aromas.

- Herbal and minty aromas blend well with citrus, earthy, and woody, and also with medicinal scents, but not so well with florals. (There's a reason you don't see many candles scented peppermint-rose.)

- Spicy aromas blend well with woody and oriental aromas.

- Oriental aromas blend well with florals. (One completely unexpected but lovely scent is a pairing of patchouli and ylang ylang.)

- Herbaceous aromas blend well with woody and citrus aromas.

- Medicinal aromas are probably the hardest to blend with other aromas, but they work with herbal and citrus essential oils.

Aromas include:

- Citrus
- Earthy
- Floral
- Herbaceous
- Medicinal
- Minty
- Oriental
- Spicy
- Woody

EIGHT REASONS TO DIY AROMATHERAPY

If you are someone who enjoys scent for the sensual experience it is, DIY aromatherapy is an enjoyable way to indulge your passion. There are many easy and fun products you can make to replace store-bought versions. But beyond that, there are a number of good reasons to add aromatherapy to your life.

1. **To reduce the amount of toxic chemicals in your home.** You know those movies where someone assembles a bomb out of a few household cleaning products or makes a flamethrower out of an aerosol spray can? There's a reason rubber gloves were invented. The chemicals in many household products cause skin irritation, and repeated inhalation of noxious fumes can cause respiratory problems. Even more important, if you have children in your home, using DIY products based on essential oils rather than synthetic substances lessens the chance of an accidental poisoning.

2. **Aromatherapy products are cost-effective.** For the cost of one bottle of brightly colored window cleaner, you can make gallons of the DIY equivalent using water, white vinegar, and the essential oil(s) of your choice. Pine- and lemon-scented cleansers and polishes can be whipped up in minutes and will make your house truly smell fresh. DIY aromatherapy products are not only cheaper than commercial products but also are often more effective, which is a win-win any day.

3. **Aromatherapy products do double (or even triple) duty.** Essential oils put the "multi" in multipurpose. Many have a whole medicine kit of properties, including analgesic, antiseptic, antispasmodic, antifungal, anti-inflammatory, and more. Lavender oil, for instance, is well known for its anxiety-soothing, sleep-inducing properties. But it also is an essential component of the disinfectant blend known as "Thieves' Oil," a combination of essential oils so powerful it was used in the Middle Ages to protect against the plague. Lavender is also an excellent ingredient for giving linens a sweet, fresh smell and adds a lovely floral scent to cosmetic products.

4. **Aromatherapy products can be a safe, nonaddictive alternative to over-the-counter medicines.** While this book does not advocate replacing traditional medicine with aromatherapy, essential oil treatments do not come with the list of side effects associated with conventional medicines: When used for headache relief, they won't cause kidney damage the way some common pain-relief remedies do. Lavender preparations to alleviate insomnia, and peppermint oil spray to sharpen focus and lift spirits will not lead to dangerous dependencies.

Moreover, if you make your own products, you know exactly what's in them.

5. **You control the quality of the products you use.** There are all sorts of sales ploys used to convince us the products we buy and use are safe, but even broad labels like "natural" can be misleading or even downright deceptive because there are no regulations about the use of similar terms. If you make your own products you know the quality of the essential oils and carrier oils you're using and you don't have to guess.

6. **Essential oils are cruelty-free.** As a conscious consumer, it's good to know that the ingredients in the products you use—particularly cosmetics—are cruelty-free. Despite years of bad press and public shaming, some mega-companies are still testing their products on animals, blinding them (and worse) in the name of beauty.

7. **You can have a "signature scent."** One scent does not fit all and even a store that stocks a wide range of cosmetics and bath products may not have a scent that draws you in. Why settle for a generic lemon scent when you can make your own Meyer lemon body scrub or a shampoo scented with blood orange instead of the more common "sweet orange" scent? Experimenting at home with oils is an affordable and fun way to create your own signature scent.

8. **Aromatherapy products make great gifts.** Homemade gifts really are the most personal way to mark an occasion and if you're on a budget, they allow you to offer the gift of luxury for pennies on the dollar. The basic ingredients for a pint of decadently desirable hand lotion, for example, can cost less than a bottle of no-name "pink" lotion from the nearest drug store. Handmade candles made with natural waxes, FDA-approved colorings for use in drugs and cosmetics (D&C), and lead-free wicks are not only fragrant and festive but also much healthier and cheaper than those pricey pillars you can buy. They might smell lovely, but who knows what you're inhaling along with the scent?

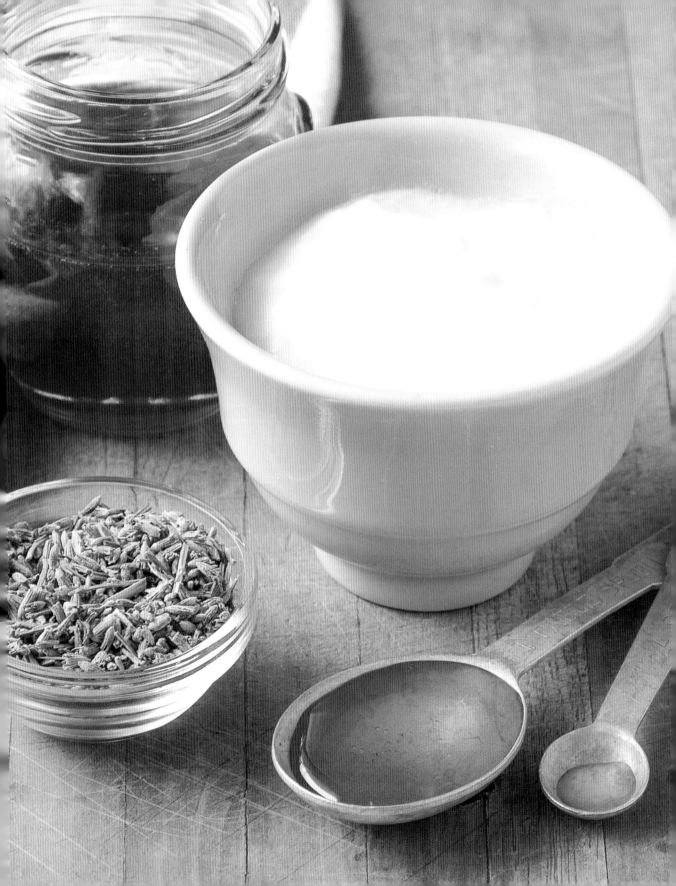

2

SHOPPING FOR AROMATHERAPY PROJECTS

Remember how exciting it used to be to shop for school supplies every fall? For an adult, embarking on a new hobby or project can bring the same sort of enthusiasm. Working with aromatherapy blends art and science in a way that satisfies creative urges such as crafting new and unique scents. It also allows you to solve practical problems, such as helping you release stress from your life. Aromatherapy has never been more popular than it is right now, especially for do-it-yourselfers. Because of this, it's easy to find the supplies you need to engage in this fun and productive hobby. Whether shopping online or in local shops, when you know where to look, you'll easily find the supplies you need.

CORE INGREDIENTS

At the heart of basic DIY aromatherapy are two core ingredients: essential oils and carrier oils. With these two ingredients you can begin basic projects, adding more items as you need them to create more complex recipes.

ESSENTIAL OILS

When selecting essential oils for projects, you need to use the best quality oils you can afford. Of course, price is not necessarily an indication of quality when it comes to essential oils. Keep the following in mind as a roadmap to evaluating the quality and versatility of the essential oils.

SCENT

Essential oils have nine basic scent categories that can help you identify the type of fragrance you'll get with each essential oil. Because essential oils come tightly sealed, you can't open the lid to smell them in the store. Knowing the basic aroma category of the essential oil will, at least from a broad perspective, give you an understanding of how the essential oil will smell. Some essential oils fall into more than one of the nine categories:

- Citrus (orange, lemon, grapefruit, bergamot, mandarin, etc.)
- Earthy (sandalwood, cypress, patchouli, black pepper, etc.)
- Floral (rose, jasmine, lavender, chamomile, ylang ylang, etc.)
- Herbaceous/Herbal (rosemary, clary sage, hyssop, basil, etc.)
- Medicinal (eucalyptus, cajeput, tea tree, etc.)
- Minty (peppermint, wintergreen, etc.)
- Oriental (ginger, patchouli, etc.)
- Spicy (cinnamon, nutmeg, ginger, clove, etc.)
- Woody (cedarwood, rosewood, pine, frankincense, etc.)

PURITY

The word "purity" as it relates to essential oils is a marketing term. Much like the label "natural," it may not have the meaning you think it does. An essential oil labeled as pure doesn't mean it is high quality or even that there is only one essential oil in the bottle. For example, it's not uncommon to find Melissa oil (also known as lemon balm) diluted with the less expensive lemon oil. In some cases, the essential oil hasn't been adulterated with another essential oil but has instead been cut with carrier oil.

One of the best ways to learn about the quality of different brands of essential oils is to do your homework before you shop. Read company literature to learn how they distill their essential oils and whether their oils are "100 percent pure" and undiluted. Look for online reviews, or talk with experienced users for recommendations of the best oils to use.

As a general rule, expect a pure essential oil to last at least a year—and many will last for more. You can find an excellent A–Z list of the approximate shelf life of popular essential oils, at www.usingeossafely.com/shelflife.

PRICE

Just as a high-priced brand doesn't necessarily indicate a high-quality essential oil, a low-priced brand may not indicate a poor-quality oil. That's why it is so important to also weigh other factors when evaluating which oils you'd like to try.

Even within one brand, prices range vastly for specific types of essential oils. Some, such as orange oil, peppermint, or tea tree oil, don't cost much to produce because the raw materials are inexpensive and easy to obtain. Others, such as jasmine and rose, require larger quantities of raw materials, or they have raw materials that are more expensive or difficult to obtain, resulting in breathtakingly high prices. Fortunately, for the very high-priced oils, you can often substitute less expensive oils that have similar properties to make your project more affordable. One great way to save money is to purchase a starter kit containing several oils from a reputable company, such as Mountain Rose Herbs.

MARKETING CLAIMS

Essential oil manufacturers use a lot of buzzwords as marketing hooks. While they may sound exciting, they don't provide meaningful descriptions of the products. Aromatherapist Jade Shutes has written extensively about the false marketing concept of "therapeutic grade" and has pointed out that claims of an essential oil being "certified" are essentially nothing more than marketing lingo. There is no official governing body that certifies essential oils or issues grades. If a brand of essential oils claims that its oils are "more therapeutic than others," you can be sure that they're exaggerating for effect.

Something else to consider when purchasing essential oils is that there is a lot of hype surrounding the oils' beneficial properties. While solid scientific evidence does exist showing the efficacy of many essential oils, be wary of extraordinary claims, which are most likely marketing hype.

BRAND REPUTATION

The Internet is a wonderful and powerful tool that allows you to do something that wasn't easily available to generations past. When used properly, the Internet can help you discover how users feel about the quality of available products and brands. This is as true for essential oils as it is for any other product on the market.

It's up to you to do your due diligence on a brand. Look for brand reviews on sites that have user-driven content. Research people's praise and concerns about each brand. It's best to look at the reviews of consensus—those reviews in which multiple parties agree. While you should certainly take into account praises and criticisms, realize that those making wildly positive or wildly negative claims may need to be given less weight—unless the bulk of customers and users make those extremely positive or negative reviews.

CARRIER OILS

With just a few exceptions, essential oils need to be diluted before they are applied to the skin or inhaled. Most commonly, they are combined with carrier oils, although you may also dilute them in alcohol, gels, and liquid soap, or add them to water for specific projects.

Carrier oils come in a wide variety of weights and prices. One of the most affordable and readily available carrier oils is olive oil, but its strong fragrance isn't ideal for use in formulas with delicate scents. Fortunately, plenty of other options exist, including plain old (inexpensive) safflower oil, which you can find near the salad dressing in any supermarket.

FROM THE MASTERS

**LEA HARRIS, CERTIFIED CLINICAL AROMATHERAPIST
AND CERTIFIED HERBALIST**

www.usingeossafely.com

One of my first experiences with essential oils that I was able to not write off as a coincidence was the success of my Bug Bite Soother.

Living in the mountains of New Hampshire, we can get some seriously big mosquitoes. We often joke that the mosquito should be our state bird. Bites would've been bad enough, but my kids were getting welts, and some scarred due to the kids' uncontrollable urge to scratch until they drew blood. I knew I had to come up with a solution.

Armed with my aromatherapy training, I made a simple blend that, to this day, is a staple in our home. It is a higher dilution than I normally use when creating a recipe, but with good reason—bug bites can cause an inflammatory response that can be quite distressing, to say the least. My formula is a blend of 50 percent carrier oil (jojoba and almond are two of many choices) and equal parts tea tree and lavender essential oils to equal the other 50 percent of the recipe. I like to combine this blend into a roller bottle for easy application.

I remember how amazed I was at how quickly the itching went away—and never to return! No more incessant scratching. No more scars. No more waking from sleep by the burn of an itch. We learned it was most effective to apply as soon as we noticed a bite. If we waited, then sometimes a second application was necessary a few hours after the first application.

My Bug Bite Soother is such an easy remedy for such a common problem. If you're just getting started with essential oils, I encourage you to give it a try.

Six of the most affordable and versatile carrier oils are:

1. **Grapeseed oil, which is particularly good for those with sensitive skin because it's naturally nonallergenic.** Because it is so affordable, it is also great for use in large quantities, such as for massage therapy. Grapeseed oil has a shelf life of between 6 and 12 months. Refrigeration may make it last a bit longer.

2. **Sweet almond oil is practical for all skin types and has a light, nutty odor that does not conflict with most blends.** It works well as a massage blend, or in some cosmetic applications. It is extremely affordable and has a shelf-life (unrefrigerated) of about 12 months.

3. **Rosehip seed oil is considered a dry oil because it absorbs in the skin so quickly.** It's not great for massage, but is wonderful in cosmetic applications for dry and aging skin, but not for acne-prone skin. It is more expensive and more perishable than some of the other carrier oils. Rosehip oil needs to be refrigerated because of its propensity to rancidity, and it lasts about 3 months, so buy it in small quantities if you plan to use it. Don't use it if you have oily skin.

4. **Apricot kernel oil is reasonably affordable and great for dry or very dry skin.** It works well in cosmetic applications. It is high in essential fatty acids and contains vitamins A and E, which are wonderful antioxidants for mature skin. Because of its light peach color, it may stain clothing.

It has a shelf life of about 12 months and doesn't require refrigeration.

5. **Jojoba oil is unique in that it is a carrier oil that remains shelf stable for a very long time—2 to 3 years in most cases.** The skin also absorbs it very well, so it's great for cosmetic use.

6. **Coconut oil has its own, relatively strong coconut fragrance.** However, because it is a solid at room temperature, it's wonderful for creating salves. To use it with essential oils, you need to melt it and mix in the essential oils, and then allow it to return to a solid at room temperature. It is shelf stable for 2 to 3 years, and works well in cosmetic and alternative health applications.

Other carrier oil options include:

ARGAN OIL is derived from the fruit of a tree native to Morocco and is used for deeply hydrating nail, skin, and hair treatments. It is expensive and should only be used for highly fragranced formulas because its own natural scent is strong.

AVOCADO OIL is a thick oil with superior skin-nourishing and moisturizing properties. It does not have a particularly long shelf life, however, so make small batches of any product that contains this oil.

CASTOR OIL is a thick oil that has antibacterial, antifungal, and antiviral properties. It works well in preparations like balms and salves that need a little "heft" to them. Castor oil should not be taken internally but, applied topically, the oil softens skin, eases inflammation, and helps heal boils, carbuncles, and abscesses.

HAZELNUT OIL is slightly astringent, which makes it a good choice for use on oily skin. It is deeply penetrating and makes a good carrier oil for massage blends. It has a naturally nutty aroma that blends well with oriental, spicy, and nutty essential oil aromas.

MACADAMIA NUT OIL is extremely regenerative and protective of the skin. It is highly absorbent and particularly suited for use on aging skin. It is used as a substitute for mink oil in the production of medicine, cosmetics, and insect repellents.

WALNUT OIL is readily available in the oils section of any supermarket. It works well as a massage oil as well as combined with other carrier oils in cosmetic products. It is consumed internally for its antioxidant properties and subtle flavor and has a strong scent.

ESSENTIAL EQUIPMENT

Just as you can prepare a delicious meal with only one pan and a single spoon, you don't really need a lot of specialized equipment to start DIY aromatherapy. All you need to make a batch of bath salts, for instance, is a measuring cup, a bowl, and a spoon. It's nice to have a pretty jar to store the final product in, but in a pinch, you could actually use almost any airtight container, even a zip-top bag. Part of the fun of working with essential oils is the aromatic alchemy of it, and for that, it's nice to have a few little extras.

PREP EQUIPMENT

When working with essential oils, you are often using precise measurements and sometimes you need to put liquids into bottles with very small mouths. You can use the food preparation equipment you already have on hand, but if you plan to do a lot of aromatherapy work, you may wish to have some dedicated glass, ceramic, or stainless steel equipment that won't be affected (or affect) the essential oils. When working with the equipment, make sure it is clean and dry before starting. Some of the following items will help you prep your essential oil formulas:

- Glass, ceramic, or metal bowls for mixing
- Glass or metal saucepan for melting and mixing
- Glass or metal stirrers, which provide a nonporous method of stirring
- Eyedroppers or pipettes for measuring oils
- Measuring spoons
- Measuring cups or scoops

- Glass liquid measuring cups for measuring carrier oils, water, and other ingredients
- Funnels to transfer products into small-mouthed storage containers
- Latex gloves to keep pure essential oils from directly contacting skin

It may also be nice to have:

- A blender for mixing large batches of liquids like hand lotion or shampoo
- A food scale for weighing small amounts of ingredients
- A candy thermometer, especially for making candles
- Protective eye goggles to prevent the concentrated essential oils from accidentally getting in your eyes

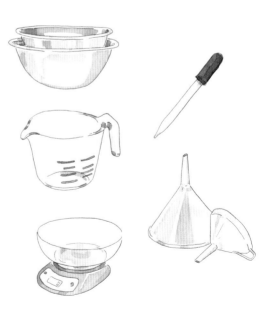

Aromatherapy prep equipment (clockwise from top left): mixing bowls, eyedropper, funnels, food scale, liquid measuring cup

STORAGE EQUIPMENT

While sometimes you make a single batch, more frequently you make a multi-use batch that requires storage items. This requires a bunch of bottles, tubs, and jars. Consider keeping on hand the following:

- Small (1- to 2-ounce) dark-colored glass roller bottles with a screw cap
- Small (4- to 8-ounce) dark-colored glass spray bottles
- Small (1- to 8-ounce) dark-colored glass jars with screw caps
- Clean mason jars

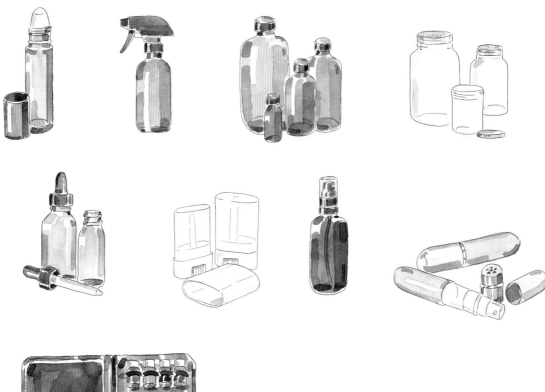

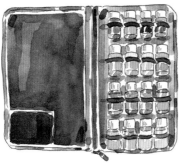

Aromatherapy equipment: (top row) glass roller bottle, glass spray bottle, glass jars with screw caps, mason jars; (middle row) screw cap dropper jars, push-up deodorant containers, glass atomizer, aluminum inhalers; (bottom row) storage container for essential oils and formulas

- Small (1 dram to 8-ounce) dark-colored screw cap dropper jars
- Empty push-up deodorant containers
- Dark-colored glass atomizers for inhaled formulas
- Aluminum inhalers (with glass inside) for inhaled formulas
- Storage container for essential oils and formulas, such as a dark box or a portfolio

When it comes to dark-colored glass, keep in mind that amber and green bottles provide the best protection from ultraviolet (UV) light. Cobalt (blue)-colored bottles are not as effective in preventing light from passing through the bottle, and through your oil as a result.

ODDS AND ENDS

You may need other items for making different products:

- Candles—wicks, and chopsticks or pencils for holding wicks
- Bath salts—wooden scoops
- All products—labels, and cute labels to make aromatherapy gifts

BOTTLES, JARS, DROPPERS, AND MORE: WHERE TO BUY EVERYTHING YOU NEED

You can get many of the basic items you need at a well-stocked grocery, drug, or home store. Some items, such as droppers and pipettes, however, may require a bit more searching.

- Amazon.com is a great one-stop shop for aromatherapy items. There, you can find pipettes, droppers, roller bottles, spray bottles, and a host of other items that may be helpful for your DIY projects.

- Another good source for droppers and pipettes, which allow for more precise measuring of your oils, is Ananda Apothecary, online at www.anandaapothecary.com.

- For self-care items, try a beauty supply store, such as Sally Beauty Supply, which is available online and in brick and mortar stores.

- A great site to buy containers in bulk is at Bulk Apothecary, www.bulkapothecary.com.

See the guide at the back of the book for a list of resources and for additional information and sources for specialized equipment.

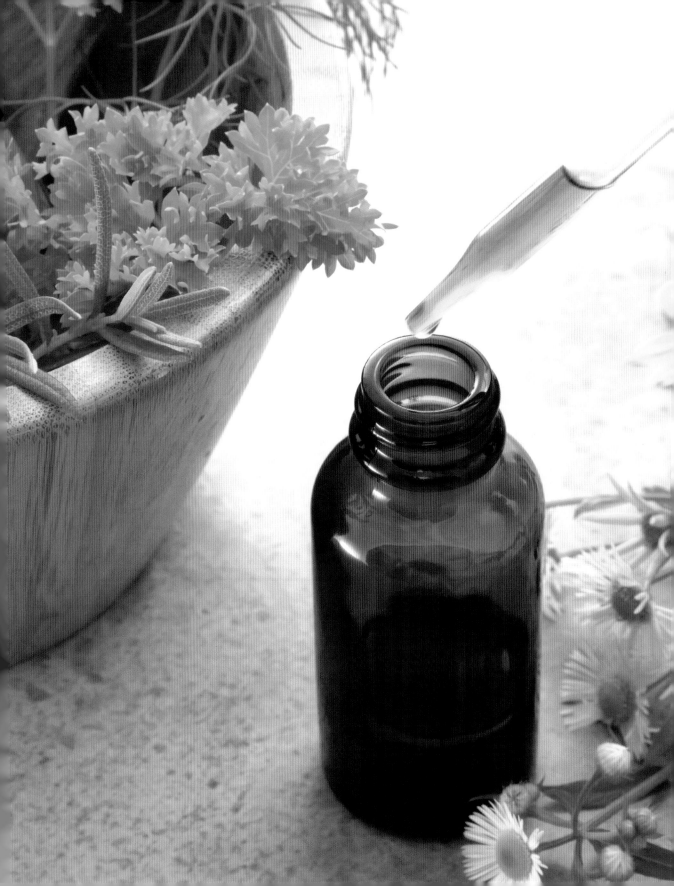

3

YOUR FIRST AROMATHERAPY BLENDS

Y ou don't have to buy an entire portfolio with hundreds of essential oils and carrier oils—or even all of the 35 oils outlined in chapter 4—to get started. In fact, with just a few different oils, you can make some fun recipes that use just one or two oils and have powerful properties, smell great, and will whet your appetite for making aromatherapy a regular part of your life.

The three recipes in this chapter are your introduction to using some of the most popular essential oils. Even if you're extremely new to aromatherapy, the projects are easy, fun, and an affordable way to enter the wonderful world of aromatherapy.

FIVE OILS AND THREE BLENDS

Swiss Army knives are incredibly popular tools because of their versatility. With a single tool, you can perform numerous functions. Consider the five oils and three blends contained in this section as your Swiss Army knife of aromatherapy. With them, you can create an array of products that work well and smell amazing.

Many manufacturers sell their essential oils in kits, and if you do some research you'll discover that these basic kits often contain the same five or six essential oils or blends. The kits are a great way to save a little bit of money and get started with essential oil blends. They typically use the same handful of oils or blends because these have powerful healing properties and are the most useful and versatile in aromatherapy work. Your five go-to oils are listed below with brief descriptions, and one or more of them are included in the three starter projects that follow. For more in-depth descriptions, please see chapter 4.

1. **Eucalyptus essential oil** works as an expectorant, and it has antibacterial and antiviral qualities. It is also cooling and soothing.

Because of this, it is incredibly versatile, helping with an array of ailments such as the common cold, muscle aches and pains, and even as an insect repellent.

2. **Lavender essential oil** not only smells great with its classic floral scent but also has a number of properties including stress release and relaxation. It's useful to help people sleep, and it has antiseptic properties making it useful for treating illness and infection.

3. **Lemon essential oil** has a delicious sunny smell, and it has powerful antibacterial properties. The citrusy smell can invigorate you and help focus your mind or soothe frayed nerves.

4. **Peppermint essential oil** has antispasmodic properties that can soothe an upset stomach. It is also an antiseptic and anti-inflammatory substance, and the smell is invigorating and helps improve focus and concentration.

5. **Tea tree essential oil** is a workhorse around the house. It has antimicrobial and antiseptic properties, and it boosts immune function. It's also great for fighting a number of common complaints including dandruff and athlete's foot.

Now feel free to dive into your first aromatherapy project. The options on the following pages include a lip balm, a disinfectant, and a candle.

THE BUZZ ON BEESWAX

To make ointments, body butters, solid perfumes, and candles, you will need beeswax, which makes a far superior base than mineral oil–based products or petroleum jelly. Natural beeswax is yellowish in color and is preferable to white beeswax, which has been bleached, or beeswax absolute, which has been treated with alcohol.

Naturally fragrant beeswax has a low melting point (around 145°F) and will discolor if over-heated. Melting beeswax in a double boiler (or in a bowl over a saucepan with simmering water) is the best method, especially if you are processing a large amount of wax.

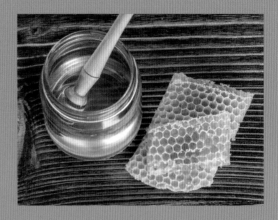

Beeswax comes in sheets, blocks of varying weights, wafers, pellets, chips, and in granules. Many recipes in this book call for grated beeswax, which requires that you grate a block or sheet yourself. In general, it costs about $1 to $1.50 an ounce, which makes beeswax one of the most inexpensive ingredients you can use in aroma-therapy projects.

Beeswax candles require more coloring than candles made with other waxes. Note too that when using golden (unprocessed) beeswax, the color of the wax will interact with any dye you might add. A dark blue dye will result in a green candle, for instance.

LEMON-PEPPERMINT LIP BALM

SCENT: MINTY/CITRUS COST: $

MAKES: 1 OUNCE

At one point or another, most people experience chapped lips. In this friendly starter recipe, just four ingredients work together to moisturize, soothe, and heal. The lemon and peppermint essential oils give this balm a sweet taste, while working as antibacterial agents to keep lips healthy and clean. Be sure to have your tins or tubes at the ready before you begin to prepare this recipe—the wax and oil mixture hardens quickly.

TIP

This lip balm recipe is infinitely customizable, and the small lip balms make great stocking stuffers and small gifts. Standard size lip balm tube containers hold roughly 0.15 ounce of balm, so this recipe will fill 6 tubes with a bit left over. Lip balm pots and tins come in a variety of sizes, with the most standard being ¼ ounce and ½ ounce. If you find that you prefer a harder texture for your lip balm than this basic recipe makes, double the amount of beeswax the next time.

3 teaspoons grated beeswax

3 teaspoons coconut oil

5 drops lemon essential oil

5 drops peppermint essential oil

1. Fill a small saucepan with a few inches of water and set it on the stove over low heat. Place a metal or glass bowl over the pan so that it fits well.

2. Add the beeswax to the bowl and wait until it melts. Then add in the coconut oil and stir to mix.

3. Remove the bowl from the heat and add the lemon and peppermint essential oils to the beeswax and oil mixture.

4. Using glass droppers or a glass liquid measuring cup (such as Pyrex), transfer the mixture to about 6 lip balm tubes or 2 to 4 tins, depending on size. Allow it to cool and harden before putting on the lid or lids.

APPLICATION: Using your finger, smooth a small amount on your lips as needed, 3 or 4 times per day.

STORAGE: Store the tightly closed jar in a cool, dry place for up to 12 months.

LAVENDER MOISTURIZING HAND CREAM

SCENT: FLORAL COST: $

MAKES: 3 OUNCES

Egyptians used hand and body lotions scented with all manner of herbs and spices, but surprisingly, there's evidence that even 12,000 years ago, ancient humans were rubbing the oil from castor plants onto their skin. Use this hand cream throughout the day to fight dryness from washing your hands, weather, and other activities.

TIP

Another 6 tablespoons of carrier oil can be added before stirring in the essential oil to make this more of a lotion than a cream.

1 ounce cocoa butter
1 ounce beeswax
2 tablespoons sweet almond oil
20 drops lavender essential oil

1. Fill a small saucepan with a few inches of water and set it on the stove over low heat. Place a metal or glass bowl over the pan so that it fits well.

2. Add the cocoa butter and beeswax to the bowl and wait until the beeswax melts.

3. Remove the bowl from the heat and add the sweet almond oil, mixing well.

4. Stir in the lavender essential oil with a metal spoon or glass stirring rod.

5. Transfer the mixture to a 3-ounce bottle or jar, and allow it to cool and harden before putting on the lid.

APPLICATION: Smooth a small amount over the front and back of hands as needed throughout the day.

STORAGE: Store in a tightly sealed container. If you carry it in your purse, the cream will last for 6 months. If the cream is stored in a cool, dark location, it will last for as long as 12 months.

FIVE THIEVES' DISINFECTANT SPRAY

SCENT: MEDICINAL/CITRUS COST: $

MAKES: 3 OUNCES

This powerful antibacterial spray was inspired by the legend of the "Thieves' Oil," a tale that dates back to the Middle Ages where it was said thieves robbing the dead protected themselves against the Black Death by washing their hands in water (or vinegar) treated with these fragrant essential oils. The legend may or may not be true, but every one of the essential oils in this recipe has potent antiseptic properties. If it could prevent the spread of plague, think what it can do against a cold germ.

1½ ounces distilled water
1½ ounces unflavored vodka
10 drops lemon essential oil
5 drops eucalyptus essential oil
5 drops lavender essential oil
5 drops tea tree essential oil

1. In a 4-ounce bottle with a spray top, add the water and vodka, and shake to mix.

2. Add the lemon, eucalyptus, lavender, and tea tree essential oils, and shake again.

APPLICATION: Spray on the surface to be cleaned and wipe away with a paper or cloth towel.

STORAGE: Store in the spray bottle, tightly sealed, in a cool, dry location for up to 12 months.

FIVE COMMON AROMATHERAPY MISTAKES

There aren't that many hard and fast rules in the world of DIY aromatherapy. There are some common-sense guidelines—don't walk away from the stove when you're melting beeswax, for example—but by and large, no one's standing over you like an Olympic ice skating judge who saw every mistake you made on that triple toe-loop. Even so, when beginning any new venture, mistakes are likely to be made. Familiarizing yourself ahead of time with some of the most common aromatherapy missteps can help you to avoid making them in the first (or at least second) place.

MISTAKE #1: USING UNDILUTED OILS

Aromatherapy oils are so concentrated that they can irritate the skin, cause photosensitivity reactions, or build up in the body and lead to a sensitization response. Always dilute essential oils. If you get undiluted essential oils on your skin, wash them away with soap and water immediately.

MISTAKE #2: USING TOO MUCH ESSENTIAL OIL

Some people want their products to have a strong scent, so they use more essential oils than a recipe calls for. While this may make the end product more fragrant, it might also irritate the skin or nasal passages. It's important to follow recipes exactly. When you have gained experience and confidence with essential oils and are beginning to make your own recipes, the rule to follow is: Use no more than one drop of essential oil per teaspoon of carrier oil.

MISTAKE #3: USING POROUS MATERIALS FOR MIXING, MEASURING, AND POURING

Porous materials like plastic will absorb fragrance. Once those aromas are there, they are there to stay, which can muddle the fragrances of future recipes made with the same objects. If you use plastic stirrers, funnels, droppers, or pipettes, consider them single-use objects. For mixing, use glass or metal bowls and stirring rods, and use metal funnels or dispose of plastic funnels after a single use.

MISTAKE #4: STORING IMPROPERLY

Essential oils are volatile and break down over time. Most manufacturers put them in dark glass jars, which keeps the light out and preserves the oils. Still, in order to preserve the oils for as long as possible, store the bottles tightly sealed in a cool, dry location away from a heat source or vibration, both of which can break down the volatile compounds more quickly.

MISTAKE #5: BUYING TOO MANY OILS

Getting started with essential oils is exciting and fun, so it's easy to get carried away. Don't purchase the biggest starter kit you can find, because it may be difficult to use all of those oils before they go bad. Instead, buy a few commonly used starter oils such as lavender, peppermint, and lemon, and then add a few more as needed. Check the oils after about six months and again after a year to ensure they remain fresh, and discard those with an off scent.

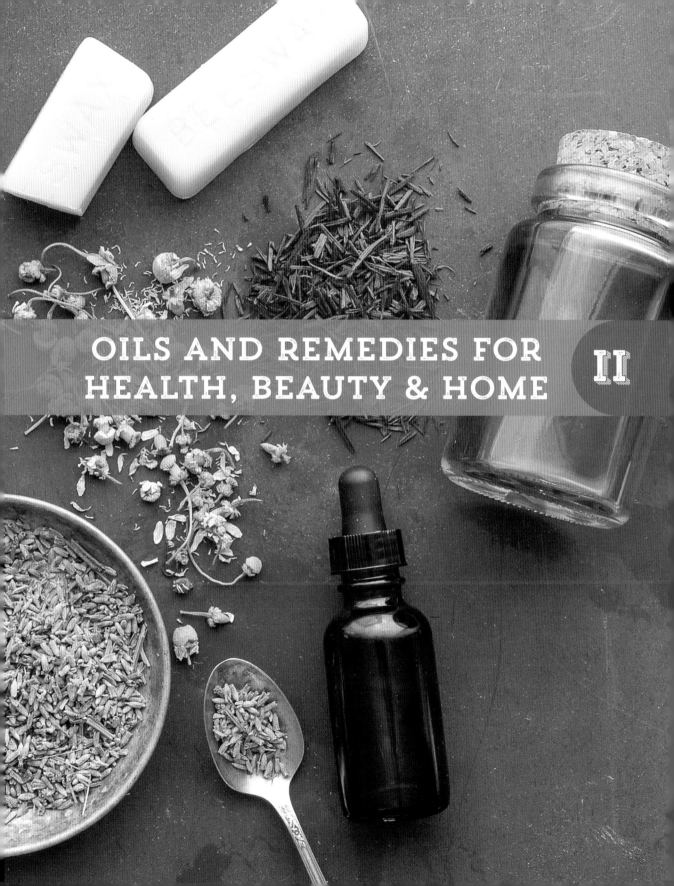

OILS AND REMEDIES FOR HEALTH, BEAUTY & HOME

II

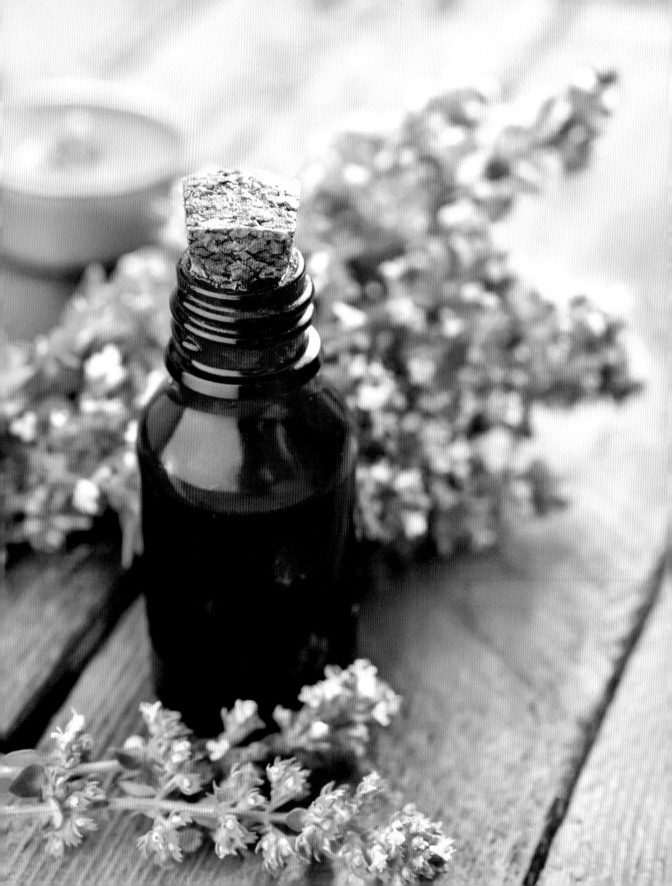

4

35 OILS TO KNOW AND USE

There are hundreds of essential oils and blends available for your DIY needs, but knowing which one suits your needs can take a little research. If you're interested in making your own nontoxic baby lotions, for example, you need to know which oils are safe for infants (lavender and dill, for instance) and, more importantly, which are not (rosemary, eucalyptus).

Just as you wouldn't treat a headache with a spoon of cough syrup, it makes sense to focus on the oils that fit the specific requirement of your project—whether it's making an antiseptic salve, a nourishing eye cream, or a disinfectant spray to remove pet odors.

COST KEY

The following pages contain the profiles of the most common, affordable, and useful essential oils available. For each essential oil, a cost rating is included.

$	$1 to $9
$$	$10 to $20
$$$	$21 to $35

This rating is based on the price of ½ ounce (15 mL) of essential oil. There are approximately 300 drops of essential oil in ½ ounce, and most recipes only use a few drops, so ½ ounce should last a while unless you're crafting blends on a large scale.

Some essential oils may cost as much as $35 for a 15 mL bottle (hops flower, helichrysum, and rose, for example), but there are plenty of great-smelling, equally therapeutic essential oils that work for DIY projects and won't stress your budget.

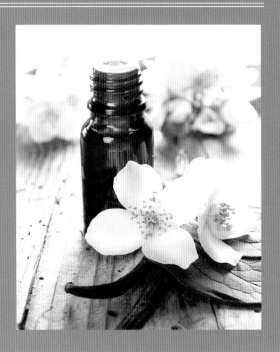

BASIL

Ocimum basilicum

SCENT: HERBACEOUS/SPICY   NOTE: TOP   COST: $

Native to India, where it is considered sacred, basil is widely used in Ayurvedic medicine. The herb has also been used in funerary rites since ancient times and is commonly planted on graves in ancient Persia, Malaysia, and Greece. Egyptians believed the leaves opened the gates of heaven and in ancient India, sprigs of the herb were placed in the hands of the dead to ease their passage to the next world. The Romans used it to treat wounds, mixing it with honey to make an antiseptic salve.

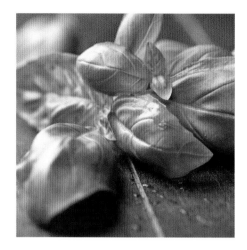

PROPERTIES
Antibacterial, Antidepressant, Anti-inflammatory, Antiseptic, Antispasmodic

POTENTIAL USES
Abrasions, Acne, Brain fog, Cleaning products, Digestive issues, Gout, Insect bites and stings, Loss of appetite, Menstrual cramps, Muscle aches, Respiratory problems

BLENDS WELL WITH
Citrus: lemon, lemongrass, lime, grapefruit, orange, neroli
Herbal: thyme, parsley
Floral: lavender, clary sage, chamomile

CAN BE SUBSTITUTED WITH
Oregano
Thyme

PRECAUTIONS
Avoid use while pregnant or breastfeeding.
Avoid use if you suffer from epilepsy.

BERGAMOT

Citrus bergamia

SCENT: CITRUS/FLORAL   NOTE: TOP   COST: $$

Bergamot oil is used both in food preparation and perfumery. It is the oil that gives Earl Grey tea its distinctive taste. It has also been used to flavor pipe tobacco. The best bergamot oil is sourced from Italy, although the plant also grows in Africa, southern France, and parts of Turkey, where it is primarily used to flavor marmalade. It is some-times adulterated with the essential oil of bergamot mint.

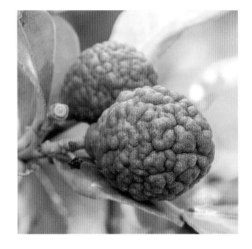

PROPERTIES

Antidepressant, Antifungal, Antiseptic, Deodorant, Digestive tonic, Febrifuge, Immune booster, Insect repellent, Sedative

POTENTIAL USES

Acne, Anxiety, Body odor, Colds and flu, Cold sores, Cough, Depression, Digestive problems, Dry Skin, Eczema, Fever, Insomnia, Laryngitis, Mood disorders, Nerve pain, Psoriasis, Scabies, Seborrhea, Skin infection, Skin irritation, Stress and tension, Urinary tract infections, Wound healing

BLENDS WELL WITH

Citrus: grapefruit, orange, bergamot
Floral: lavender, geranium, palmarosa, ylang ylang
Oriental: patchouli
Spicy: cinnamon, clove, nutmeg

CAN BE SUBSTITUTED WITH

Bitter Orange
Grapefruit

PRECAUTIONS

Never use more than 1 drop per 2 teaspoons of carrier oil.
Do not spend time in the sun after using this essential oil.

BLACK PEPPER

Piper nigrum

SCENT: SPICY/WOODY **NOTE:** MIDDLE **COST:** $$

Black pepper is the most widely used spice in the world. The plant is native to India, but Vietnam is now the world's largest producer and exporter of the spice, which is derived from the dried fruit (the peppercorn) of the plant. In arcane herbcraft, black pepper was used to banish negativity and ward off petty jealousy. Perfumes scented with black pepper include Fleur Poivrée by Acorelle, Aurien Nigra by Eudora, and Popy Moreni.

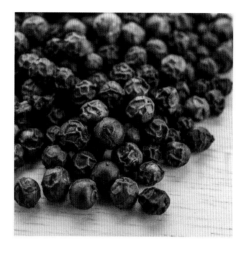

PROPERTIES

Analgesic, Antibacterial, Digestive tonic, Febrifuge , Improves circulation, Strengthens immunity, Thermogenic

POTENTIAL USES

Arthritis, Digestive issues, Fever, Menstrual cramps, Muscle aches and cramps, Muscle strain, Nerve pain, Poor circulation

BLENDS WELL WITH

Citrus: bergamot, grapefruit, orange, lemon
Floral: ylang ylang, geranium
Herbal: basil, thyme, rosemary
Oriental: patchouli, frankincense
Spicy: nutmeg, cinnamon
Woody: cypress, sandalwood

CAN BE SUBSTITUTED WITH

Coriander

PRECAUTIONS

Avoid use while pregnant or breastfeeding.
Avoid use if you suffer from kidney or liver disease.

CALENDULA

Calendula officinalis

SCENT: FLORAL   NOTE: MIDDLE   COST: $$

Also known as the pot marigold, calendula is one of the few flowers that produces an essential oil and not an absolute. The flower has a long history of being associated with sacred rituals and was used to adorn Hindi temples, and revered by the Egyptians for its regenerative properties. Calendula ointments have long been used to treat conjunctivitis (pink eye) and as a gentle lotion for diaper rash.

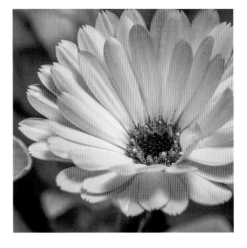

PROPERTIES
Anti-inflammatory, Antispasmodic, Sedative, Skincare, Soporific, Tonic

POTENTIAL USES
Acne, Anxiety, Burns, Cold sores, Menstrual issues, Psoriasis, Skin irritation

BLENDS WELL WITH
Citrus: orange, lemon, neroli
Floral: lavender, chamomile
Woody: cypress, pine, cedarwood

CAN BE SUBSTITUTED WITH
Lavender

PRECAUTIONS
Avoid use if pregnant or breastfeeding.

CEDARWOOD

Juniperus virginiana

SCENT: WOODY   NOTE: BASE   COST: $

The scent of cedarwood is said to have a grounding, calming effect. The ancient Romans and Greeks burned the wood to scent the air. It was nick-named the "Tree of Life" (*arborvitae*). It is used for fencing and roofing. The wood's scent is a natural moth repel-lent and chests made of the fragrant wood were often used to store clothes. Increasingly, the wood is also being used for "green" coffins.

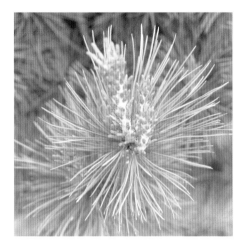

PROPERTIES
Antibacterial, Antifungal, Antiseptic, Astringent (mild), Decongestant, Insecticide, Sedative

POTENTIAL USES
Acne, Arthritis, Cold/flu, Cough, Dermatitis, Eczema, Fungal infections, Insect repellent, Oily skin, Psoriasis, Skin conditions, Urinary tract infections

BLENDS WELL WITH
Citrus: bergamot, lemon
Floral: lavender
Herbal: rosemary
Woody: cypress

CAN BE SUBSTITUTED WITH
Cypress

PRECAUTIONS
Avoid use while pregnant or breastfeeding.
Some sources cite cedarwood as an abortifacient, while others claim it is safe to use in pregnancy.

CHAMOMILE

Chamaemelum nobile (Roman Chamomile)
Matricaria recutita (German Chamomile)

SCENT: FLORAL   NOTE: TOP   COST: $$

Chamomile is moderately priced, but it's well worth the few extra dollars it costs for this versatile and gentle essential oil. Typically, you'll find two varieties of chamomile: Roman and German. You can use these two oils interchangeably in preparations and recipes. Chamomile is related to ragweed, so people with a ragweed allergy may be sensitive to topical application of chamomile.

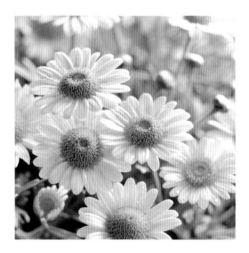

PROPERTIES

Antibacterial, Antifungal, Anti-inflammatory, Calming, Digestive tonic, Numbs nerve pain, Stimulates bile production, Stimulates urine flow

POTENTIAL USES

Abrasions, Arthritis, Cold sores, Colic, Dermatitis, Diarrhea, Digestive upset, Dry skin, Eczema, Fungal infections, Gas, Headache, Hives, Inflammation, Insect bites, Insomnia, Menstrual problems, Migraine, Nerve pain, Premenstrual symptoms, Sprains and strains, Stomach upset, Stress, Teething, Toothache, Urinary tract infection, Wound healing

BLENDS WELL WITH

Floral: geranium, rose, lavender
Oriental: patchouli

CAN BE SUBSTITUTED WITH

Lavender

PRECAUTIONS

May interact with certain drugs. Talk to your doctor or pharmacist about potential interactions.

CINNAMON (BARK OR LEAF)

Cinnamomum zeylancium

SCENT: SPICY   **NOTE:** BASE TO MIDDLE   **COST:** $$$

Cinnamon oil is distilled from both the leaf and the bark of the cinnamon tree. Cinnamon leaf costs roughly one-fifth what cinnamon bark oil does, but you can use the two interchangeably depending on what you have available. Cinnamon is used as a spice for cooking, a flavoring for candy, dental products, and alcoholic spirits like spiced rum, whiskey, and tequila. The tree is hardy and can grow in soil that is 99 percent pure sand.

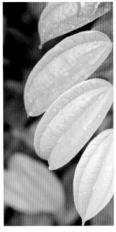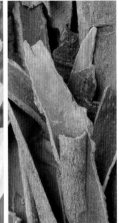

PROPERTIES
Antibacterial, Antidepressant, Antifungal, Anti-inflammatory, Antimicrobial, Antiparasitic, Antiseptic, Astringent (mild), Insecticide, Thermogenic

POTENTIAL USES
Arthritis, Bee stings, Colds/flu, Digestive problems, Gas, Insect bites, Insect repellent, Lice, Nerve pain, Poor appetite, Stomach upset, Yeast (candida) infection

BLENDS WELL WITH

Citrus: orange, bergamot, mandarin, grapefruit
Floral: ylang ylang, lavender
Herbal: thyme
Spicy: nutmeg, ginger, clove
Woody: frankincense, pine

CAN BE SUBSTITUTED WITH

Clove

PRECAUTIONS

Avoid use while pregnant.

CLARY SAGE

Salvia sclarea

SCENT: EARTHY/FLORAL NOTE: BASE TO MIDDLE COST: $$

Native to southern Europe, clary sage essential oil has a slightly pungent, earthy odor. While it costs slightly more than other essential oils, clary sage is a good tool to have in your arsenal. It is extremely versatile for health purposes, and it is a mild oil that is safe for use with most people.

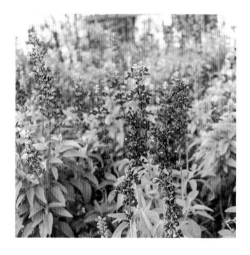

PROPERTIES
Antiseptic, Aphrodisiac, Deodorizing, Emmenagogue, Mood elevating, Muscle relaxant, Sedative, Tonic

POTENTIAL USES
Acne, Bee stings, Body odor, Cough, Dandruff, Digestive issues, Gas, High blood pressure, Insomnia, Menstrual cramps, Muscle aches and pains, Premenstrual syndrome, Sexual problems, Stress

BLENDS WELL WITH
Floral: geranium, lavender
Woody: juniper, sandalwood, cedarwood

CAN BE SUBSTITUTED WITH
Lavender

PRECAUTIONS
Avoid use while pregnant.

CLOVE

Syzygium aromaticum

SCENT: SPICY/WOODY   NOTE: MIDDLE   COST: $

Unscrupulous vendors may dilute clove oil with copaiba or pimento essential oil. In pioneer dentistry, oil of cloves was used to deaden the pain of decayed teeth and inflamed gums, but it's not recommended for internal use. It is a sacred spice and in ancient times, clove trees were planted to mark a child's birth. (It was a bad sign if the tree failed to thrive.) Cloves are used in cooking and are also smoked as a substitute for tobacco.

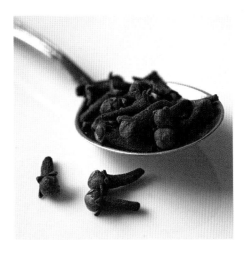

PROPERTIES

Analgesic, Antibacterial, Antiseptic, Antispasmodic, Digestive tonic, Disinfectant, Eases nerve pain, Insect repellent, Muscle relaxant

POTENTIAL USES

Acne, Arthritis, Asthma, Athlete's foot, Bad breath, Bronchitis, Burns, Cleaning products, Digestive upset, Gas, Infection, Nerve pain, Toothache

BLENDS WELL WITH

Citrus: orange, mandarin
Oriental: patchouli
Spicy: ginger, nutmeg, cinnamon

CAN BE SUBSTITUTED WITH

Cinnamon
Copaiba

PRECAUTIONS

Avoid use while pregnant.
Avoid use if suffering from liver or kidney conditions.
Avoid use in young children under the age of 3.
Dilute to no more than 1 drop per 2 teaspoons of carrier oil.
May react with certain medications. Talk to your doctor or pharmacist about potential interactions.

CORIANDER SEED

Coriandrum sativum

SCENT: SPICY   NOTE: MIDDLE   COST: $

Coriander (also known as cilantro) is used as a food flavoring and is one of the ingredients of gin. It was known to the Egyptians, Romans, Greeks, and Israelites, and an ancient Chinese legend said that eating the seeds would confer immortality. "Coriander water" is an old remedy for the "windy colic." Coriander's spicy note is part of several memorable perfumes, including Drakkar Noir by Guy Laroche, Live Jazz from Yves Saint Laurent, and Coriandre from Jean Couturier.

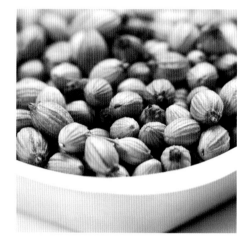

PROPERTIES

Analgesic, Antifungal, Antispasmodic, Aphrodisiac, Deodorant

POTENTIAL USES

Athlete's foot, Body odor, Dandruff, Headache, Muscle pain, Muscle spasm, Sexual problems

BLENDS WELL WITH
Citrus: bergamot, grapefruit, neroli
Floral: clary sage, ylang ylang
Spicy: black pepper, ginger
Woody: frankincense

CAN BE SUBSTITUTED WITH
Rosewood
Thyme

PRECAUTIONS
None specific

CYPRESS

Cupressus sempervirens

SCENT: WOODY/BALSAMIC NOTE: MIDDLE COST: $$

The Phoenicians and Cretans used cypress for boat building. Cypress trees have long been associated with death and funeral rites. Ancient Egyptians built coffins out of the wood. In Greek mythology, the tree was sacred to Hades, ruler of the underworld. Both Greeks and Romans planted the tree outside their temples and cemeteries. The essential oil is said to boost the effects of negative ions in the air.

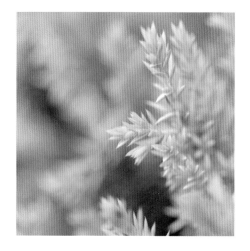

PROPERTIES
Antiseptic, Antispasmodic, Astringent (strong), Deodorant, Diuretic, Sedative, Tonic

POTENTIAL USES
Arthritis, Bleeding, Broken capillaries, Edema (swelling), Hemorrhoids, Insect repellent, Menstrual cramps, Muscle cramps/spasms, Oily skin, Poor circulation, Premenstrual syndrome, Urinary tract infection, Varicose veins, Water retention

BLENDS WELL WITH
Citrus: lime, orange, lemon, grapefruit
Floral: ylang ylang, lavender
Spicy: ginger, black pepper
Woody: benzoin, cedarwood, pine

CAN BE SUBSTITUTED WITH
Cedarwood

PRECAUTIONS
None specific

EUCALYPTUS

Eucalyptus globulus

SCENT: WOODY/MEDICINAL   **NOTE:** TOP   **COST:** $

Eucalyptus leaves are a koala bear's favorite food. There are more than 700 species of the plant, most of them native to Australia, where the indigenous people have used the plant in their medicines for centuries. It is now widely used as an inhalant to treat colds and other respiratory illnesses, and topically for muscle aches and pains. It is also used to flavor cough drops.

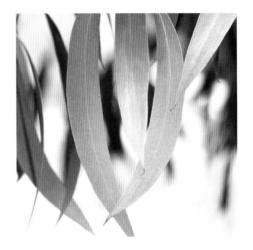

PROPERTIES

Antibacterial, Antiseptic, Antiviral, Calming, Decongestant, Expectorant, Febrifuge, Insecticide, Numbs nerves, Stain remover

POTENTIAL USES

Abrasions, Aches and pains, Arthritis, Bacterial infection, Blisters, Bronchitis, Bug spray, Burns, Cleaning products, Cold/flu, Congestion, Coughs, Fever, Urinary tract infection

BLENDS WELL WITH

Citrus: grapefruit
Floral: chamomile, geranium
Minty: peppermint
Woody: cedarwood, cypress, juniper

CAN BE SUBSTITUTED WITH

Niaouli
Tea Tree

PRECAUTIONS

Avoid use with children 10 years old or younger.

FRANKINCENSE

Boswellia carterii

SCENT: WOODY/SPICY/ORIENTAL   NOTE: BASE   COST: $$$

Long before biblical times, frankincense was known as a precious plant, burned by the Egyptians as incense and used in their perfumes. Frankincense resin is harvested by "wounding" the tree in a process known as striping. The resin that drips out then hardens and is known as "tears." The tree is extremely hardy and can even grow on solid rock. The Roman Catholic Church sources most of its frankincense from Somalia, which produces the highest-quality resin.

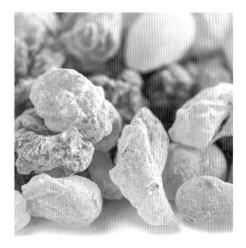

PROPERTIES

Antibacterial, Antiseptic, Astringent, Cicatrizant, Decongestant, Disinfectant, Diuretic, Sedative, Tonic

POTENTIAL USES

Abrasions, Aging skin, Asthma, Bacterial infection, Cleaning products, Congestion, Cough, Gas, Menstrual problems, Oily skin, Urinary tract infection

BLENDS WELL WITH

Citrus: orange, mandarin, lime, bergamot
Floral: lavender
Oriental: patchouli
Spicy: cinnamon

CAN BE SUBSTITUTED WITH

Myrrh

PRECAUTIONS

Avoid use while pregnant or breastfeeding.

GERANIUM

Pelargonium graveolens

SCENT: FLORAL   NOTE: MIDDLE   COST: $$

One of the few flower oils available for a reasonable price, geranium is prized for its "rosy" notes and may be sold as rose geranium. It has a calming effect both physically and mentally, and has been distilled since the early 19th century. In the 17th century, English gardeners planted the flower to protect against evil spirits. In the language of flowers, geraniums represent gentility. It is used in Ayurvedic medicine to treat menstrual and menopausal symptoms, as well as depression.

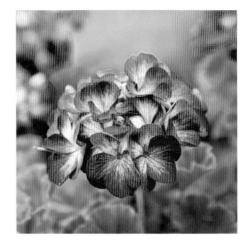

PROPERTIES
Analgesic, Antianxiety, Anti-inflammatory, Antifungal, Antiseptic, Diuretic, Hormone regulation, Numbing, Pesticide

POTENTIAL USES
Abrasions, Acne, Anxiety, Bruises, Dry skin, Dust mites, Hemorrhoids, Lice, Menopause, Menstrual problems, Nerve pain, PMS, Sore throat, Tonsilitis

BLENDS WELL WITH
Citrus: orange, lemon, bergamot
Floral: ylang ylang
Oriental: patchouli
Spicy: black pepper, cinnamon, nutmeg, clove
Woody: cypress, sandalwood

CAN BE SUBSTITUTED WITH
Palmarosa
Rose otto

PRECAUTIONS
Avoid use while pregnant.
May interact with certain medications. Talk with your doctor or pharmacist about potential interactions.

GINGER

Zingiber officinale

SCENT: SPICY/ORIENTAL   **NOTE:** MIDDLE   **COST:** $$

The ginger spice was traded as early as the first century. In the 16th century, Jamaican ginger became the first "Oriental spice" to be grown in the New World and exported back to Europe. Ginger is used to flavor food, candy, soft drinks, and wine. It is used in perfume, especially in unisex and male fragrances like Zenzero Tesori d'Oriente, and Big Pony 3 by Ralph Lauren.

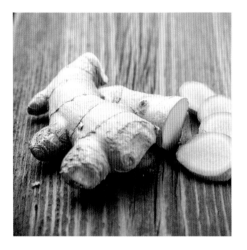

PROPERTIES
Analgesic, Anti-inflammatory, Antiseptic, Aphrodisiac, Decongestant, Digestive tonic, Febrifuge, Laxative, Thermogenic

POTENTIAL USES
Arthritis, Cold/flu, Cough, Diarrhea, Digestive issues, Fever, Gas, Heartburn, Motion sickness, Muscle aches/pains, Nausea, Pain, Sexual problems, Sore throat

BLENDS WELL WITH
Citrus: mandarin, grapefruit, lemon
Floral: ylang ylang, geranium
Oriental: patchouli, frankincense
Spicy: clove
Woody: cedarwood, juniper

CAN BE SUBSTITUTED WITH
Cardamom
Cinnamon

PRECAUTIONS
Avoid use in first trimester of pregnancy.

GRAPEFRUIT

Citrus x paradisi

SCENT: CITRUS   NOTE: TOP   COST: $

Grapefruit is believed to have originated as a hybrid between the pomelo and sweet orange sometime in the 19th century. Energy workers believe the oil is cleansing to the aura. A grapefruit half is a prop in one of the most iconic scenes in Hollywood history, the moment in *Public Enemy* when James Cagney smashes the fruit into Mae Clarke's face. Both pink and white grapefruit are used in perfumery.

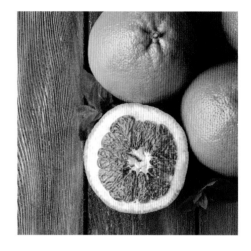

PROPERTIES
Antidepressant, Antiseptic, Detoxifying, Disinfectant, Diuretic, Stimulant, Tonic

POTENTIAL USES
Acne, Brain fog, Cleaning products, Exhaustion, Memory problems, Muscle fatigue, Muscle stiffness, Oily skin

BLENDS WELL WITH
Citrus: bergamot, orange, lemon, lime
Floral: palmarosa, ylang ylang
Herbal: rosemary
Medicinal: eucalyptus
Oriental: patchouli
Spicy: black pepper, cardamom, clove, ginger

CAN BE SUBSTITUTED WITH
Bergamot
Lemon

PRECAUTIONS
Mildly phototoxic, though the least phototoxic of the citrus oils.

JUNIPER

Juniperus communis

SCENT: WOODY   **NOTE:** MIDDLE   **COST:** $$

Juniper has been used by many cultures in purification rituals. Many modern-day energy workers use juniper essential oil to cleanse their crystals. Juniper berries lend their fragrance to gin and are also used in perfumery. Fragrances that have juniper notes include J'ai Osé Aqua by Guy Laroche, CK IN2U for Her by Calvin Klein, and Adventurer II from Eddie Bauer.

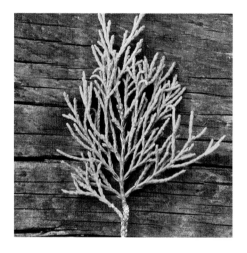

PROPERTIES
Antiseptic, Calmative, Detoxifying, Deodorant, Diuretic, Febrifuge, Insect repellent, Tonic

POTENTIAL USES
Acne, Arthritis, Body odor, Colds/flu, Dermatitis, Digestive problems, Eczema, Enlarged prostate, Fever, Fleas and ticks, Fluid retention, Food poisoning, Gout, Insects, Kidney stones, Menstrual problems, Muscular pain, Oily scalp, Oily skin, Psoriasis, Skin problems, Urinary tract infection

BLENDS WELL WITH
Earthy: oakmoss
Floral: lavender
Herbal: rosemary
Woody: cedarwood, fir needle, cypress

CAN BE SUBSTITUTED WITH
Rosemary

PRECAUTIONS
Avoid use while pregnant.
Avoid use if suffering from kidney or liver disease.

LAVENDER

Lavandula angustifolia
Lavandula latifolia (spike lavender)
Lavandula stoechas (Spanish lavender)

SCENT: FLORAL   NOTE: MIDDLE   COST: $$

Lavender is one of the oldest essential oils still in use today. The Egyptians used it in their mummification rituals and it was known to both the Greeks and Romans in classical times. In the United States, lavender is grown coast-to-coast but flourishes in the Pacific Northwest where an annual lavender festival is held in Sequim, Washington.

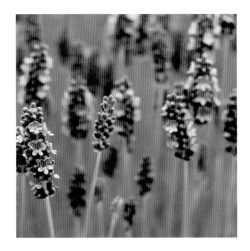

PROPERTIES

Analgesic, Antibacterial, Antifungal, Anti-inflammatory, Antiseptic, Antispasmodic, Antiviral, Insect repellent, Muscle relaxant, Stimulates cell growth

POTENTIAL USES

Abrasions, Acne, Aging skin, Anxiety, Arthritis, Athlete's foot, Bug spray, Burns, Colds/flu, Dermatitis, Eczema, Headaches, Insect bites/stings, Insomnia, Laryngitis, Menstrual cramps, Mood swings, Muscle cramping/pain, Nervous conditions, Psoriasis, Scabies, Scarring, Sciatica, Skin disorders, Sunburn

BLENDS WELL WITH

Citrus: lemon
Floral: Roman chamomile, clary sage, geranium
Spicy: nutmeg
Woody: cedarwood, pine

CAN BE SUBSTITUTED WITH

Chamomile

PRECAUTIONS

Avoid use of spike lavender and Spanish lavender if pregnant or breastfeeding.
Avoid use of spike lavender and Spanish lavender with infants and children.

LEMON

Citrus limonum

SCENT: CITRUS   **NOTE:** TOP   **COST:** $

In India, lemons are called "golden apples." Lemon essential oil is one of the most useful botanicals available to the aromatherapist. It is used for flavoring everything from pickles (popular in Asia) to candy to soda and prized for its versatility as an ingredient in cosmetics, medicinals, and nontoxic cleaning products. The fruit has an exotic heritage—born in India, given an Arabic name, and brought to Europe by the Crusaders.

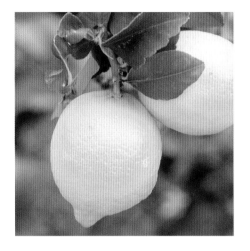

PROPERTIES
Antibacterial, Antiseptic, Astringent, Detoxification, Febrifuge, Styptic, Tonic

POTENTIAL USES
Bacterial infection, Bee stings, Bleeding, Bronchitis, Digestive upset, Fever, Headaches, Insect bites, Mouth ulcers, Muscle aches, Oily skin, Skin discoloration, Sore throat, Stain removal, Warts

BLENDS WELL WITH
Citrus: orange, mandarin, grapefruit
Earthy: oakmoss
Floral: chamomile
Herbal: fennel
Medicinal: eucalyptus, tea tree
Oriental: frankincense
Woody: benzoin, juniper, sandalwood

CAN BE SUBSTITUTED WITH
Grapefruit
Lime

PRECAUTIONS
Phototoxic if used at more than a 2 percent dilution (2 drops per teaspoon of carrier oil).

LEMONGRASS

Cymbopogon citratus (West Indian lemongrass)
Cymbopogon flexuosus (East Indian lemongrass)
SCENT: CITRUS/HERBAL **NOTE:** TOP **COST:** $

A native of Sri Lanka, this plant is used as both a culinary herb and a medicine all over Asia. It is a staple of the Ayurvedic medicine pharmacopeia, used for treating kidney infections, headaches, and depression, and also as a general tonic for the immune system. It is the source for citronella oil but "citronella" is another plant entirely. Lemongrass oil is used in waxes, polishes, detergents, and insecticides.

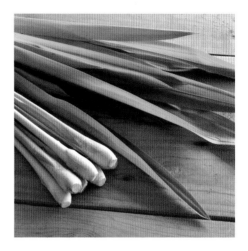

PROPERTIES

Antidepressant, Antifungal, Antiseptic, Febrifuge, Immune system strengthener, Stimulates circulation, Tonic

POTENTIAL USES

Acne, Depression, Fever, Mosquito repellent, Muscle aches, Poor circulation, Shampoo, Stress

BLENDS WELL WITH

Citrus: lemon, orange, mandarin, bergamot
Floral: lavender, geranium
Herbal: basil, thyme
Medicinal: eucalyptus, tea tree
Oriental: ginger, patchouli
Spicy: black pepper
Woody: cedarwood

CAN BE SUBSTITUTED WITH

Lemon

PRECAUTIONS

None specific

LIME

Citrus aurantifolia

SCENT: CITRUS   NOTE: TOP   COST: $

The fruit is fondly remembered as an ingredient in the nonalcoholic "Lime Rickey," which competed with a "Shirley Temple" as the go-to "cocktail" for children dining out with their parents in the 60s. The slang term "limey" for Englishmen is derived from the 18th-century practice of carrying limes on British naval ships to prevent scurvy. It is widely used as a fragrance. Perfumes with lime notes include Lime by Caswell-Massey, Old Spice Lime, and Acqua di Gio by Armani.

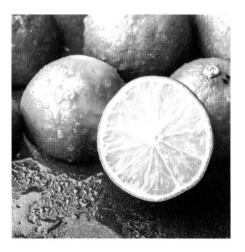

BLENDS WELL WITH

Citrus: citronella, lemon, orange, grapefruit
Floral: clary sage, lavender, neroli, ylang ylang
Herbal: rosemary
Spicy: nutmeg

CAN BE SUBSTITUTED WITH

Lemon

PRECAUTIONS

Phototoxic if used at more than a 0.7 percent dilution (4 drops per ounce).
May irritate sensitive skin.

PROPERTIES

Antiseptic, Antiviral, Astringent, Disinfectant, Febrifuge, Styptic

POTENTIAL USES

Acne, Bee stings, Bleeding, Colds/flu, Dull skin, Fever, Insect bites, Oily skin, Sore throat, Warts

MYRRH

Commiphora myrrha

SCENT: WOODY/ORIENTAL **NOTE:** BASE **COST:** $$$

An aromatic, resinous gum harvested throughout Africa, myrrh is extensively used in Chinese medicine, where it is classified as a "bitter" and "spicy" herb. In the ancient Jewish Talmud, myrrh is highly praised as a medicinal ointment, and in Muslim texts, as "balsam of Mecca." An unrelated herb called "sweet cicely" is also sometimes referred to as myrrh.

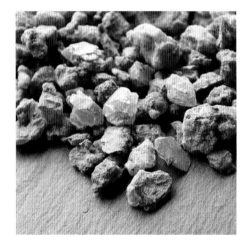

PROPERTIES
Antibacterial, Antifungal, Anti-inflammatory, Antioxidant, Cooling

POTENTIAL USES
Aging skin, Asthma, Athlete's foot, Bronchitis, Chapped skin, Colds/flu, Cough, Diarrhea, Eczema, Gas, Gingivitis, Heartburn, Inflammation, Itching, Respiratory infection, Oily skin

BLENDS WELL WITH
Citrus: bergamot
Floral: palmarosa
Minty: eucalyptus
Oriental: frankincense
Spicy: clove
Woody: sandalwood

CAN BE SUBSTITUTED WITH
Balsam

PRECAUTIONS
Avoid use while pregnant or breastfeeding.

NIAOULI

Melaleuca quinquenervia

SCENT: MEDICINAL   NOTE: MIDDLE   COST: $

Also known as the "paperbark tree," niaouli is related to the allspice family. It is native to the Pacific Island region. Like a number of nonnative plants introduced to the Everglades (Old World climbing fern, hydrilla), niaouli has become "naturalized" and the invasive plant is now threatening the area's delicate ecosystem. The oil is used as an inhalant for respiratory ailments but also heals acne, eczema, and other skin conditions.

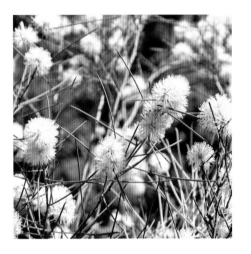

PROPERTIES
Antibacterial, Antiseptic, Decongestant, Febrifuge, Improves concentration, Numbs pain, Stimulant

POTENTIAL USES
Abrasions, Acne, Arthritis, Bad breath, Boils, Brain fog, Burns, Colds/flu, Congestion, Fever, Insect bites, Laryngitis, Muscle aches, Nerve pain, Sinusitis

BLENDS WELL WITH
Citrus: bergamot, orange, lemon
Floral: lavender
Medicinal: eucalyptus, tea tree

CAN BE SUBSTITUTED WITH
Cajeput
Tea tree

PRECAUTIONS
Avoid use in children under the age of 10.

NUTMEG

Myristica fragrans

SCENT: SPICY   **NOTE**: MIDDLE   **COST**: $$

Long used as a spice and flavoring, nutmeg is used in perfumery to fix citrus scents. It was originally used by Arab physicians (who introduced it to the Venetians) to treat digestive disorders, kidney ailments, and bad breath. Both Indians and Arabs used the spice as an aphrodisiac. The spice is mentioned in the writings of both Pliny and Hildegard of Bingen. Elizabethans used it to ward off the plague. Nutmeg is frequently used for unisex and masculine scents like Guerlain's Vetiver Sport and Dior's Fahrenheit.

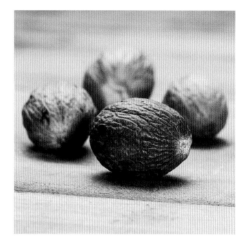

PROPERTIES

Analgesic, Anti-inflammatory, Antiseptic, Aphrodisiac, Digestive tonic, Relaxant, Sedative, Stimulant

POTENTIAL USES

Arthritis, Diarrhea, Digestive issues, Gas, Nausea, Pain, Sexual problems, Shampoo, Vomiting

BLENDS WELL WITH
Citrus: orange, grapefruit, bergamot
Earthy: oakmoss
Floral: geranium, lavender
Spicy: coriander

CAN BE SUBSTITUTED WITH
Cinnamon
Cloves

PRECAUTIONS
Avoid use while pregnant.

ORANGE

Citrus aurantium (Neroli or Bitter orange)
Citrus sinesis (Sweet orange)
Citrus reticulata (Mandarin)

SCENT: CITRUS   **NOTE:** TOP   **COST:** $

With similar scents, the essential oils in the orange family also have similar properties and can typically be substituted for one another in both health and scent formulations. Orange is used as a flavoring and also as a solvent. It is used in Ayurvedic medicine to treat gout, digestive disorders, and anxiety. Some of the perfumes that possess an orange note are Chopard's Happy Spirit and Miss Dior Cherie L'Eau by Dior.

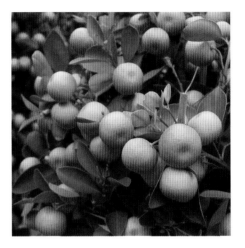

PROPERTIES
Antidepressant, Antifungal, Digestive tonic, Sedative, Skin tonic, Stimulant

POTENTIAL USES
Acne, Anxiety, Athlete's foot, Colds/flu, Depression, Fungal infections, Skin problems

BLENDS WELL WITH
Citrus: grapefruit, lemon, lime, bergamot
Floral: lavender
Spicy: black pepper, ginger

CAN BE SUBSTITUTED WITH
Grapefruit

PRECAUTIONS
Bitter orange is phototoxic.

OREGANO

Origanum vulgare

SCENT: HERBACEOUS   NOTE: MIDDLE   COST: $$

As noted in a fact sheet produced by the Herb Society of America, oregano was grown in Egypt for 3,000 years, used by the Greeks in classical times, and used by the Hittites, who lived in the area that is now Syria and who inscribed images of the herb on clay tablets. The herb is highly prized as a food flavoring, especially in Mediterranean cooking, as well as for its therapeutic qualities, which were noted by Greek physician Hippocrates.

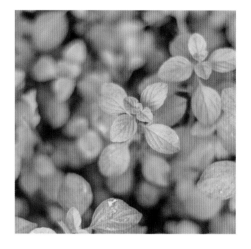

PROPERTIES

Antibacterial, Antifungal, Antiparasitic

POTENTIAL USES

Athlete's foot, Bacterial infection, Fungal infection, Intestinal parasites

BLENDS WELL WITH

Citrus: bergamot, orange, lemon
Floral: lavender
Medicinal: eucalyptus
Woody: cedarwood

CAN BE SUBSTITUTED WITH

Basil
Marjoram
Thyme

PRECAUTIONS

Avoid use while pregnant.
May inhibit blood clotting.

PALMAROSA

Cymbopogon martinii

SCENT: FLORAL   **NOTE:** MIDDLE   COST: $

Palmarosa essential oil is extracted from a flowering grass harvested before it flowers. It was used by ancient Indian doctors to treat nerve pain, rheumatism, and infectious diseases. It is valued as a perfume ingredient because of the "rosy note" in its aroma. Alternate names for palmarosa include Turkish rose, Indian rose, and rose geranium. Perfumes with palmarosa notes include Ciara by Revlon and Jasmin 17 by Le Labo.

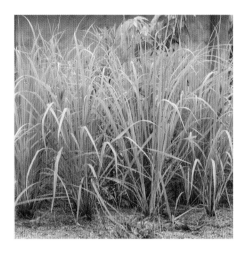

PROPERTIES
Antibacterial, Anti-inflammatory, Antiseptic, Antiviral, Appetite stimulant, Febrifuge, Insect repellent, Stimulates cell growth

POTENTIAL USES
Abrasions, Aches and pains, Acne, Aging skin, Bacterial infection, Dermatitis, Eczema, Gastroenteritis, Psoriasis, Rosacea, Scarring, Skin irritation

BLENDS WELL WITH
Citrus: orange, bergamot
Oriental: patchouli
Floral: ylang ylang
Herbal: rosemary
Woody: amyris, cedarwood, sandalwood

CAN BE SUBSTITUTED WITH
Geranium
Rose

PRECAUTIONS
May interact with certain medications. Talk to your doctor or pharmacist about potential interactions.

PATCHOULI

Pogostemon cablin

SCENT: EARTHY/SPICY   **NOTE**: BASE   **COST**: $$

If the 1970s were a person, patchouli oil would have been her signature scent. It is used in Chinese traditional medicines and also in Wiccan rituals, where it substitutes for graveyard dust. It is highly prized for its skin-conditioning properties and used to treat eczema, rashes, acne, chapped skin, and dermatitis. Its use in perfumery is widespread, with scents as different as Lorenzo Villoresi's Patchouli, Sergei Lutens' Borneo 1834, and Angel by Thierry Mugler demonstrating how subtle patchouli can be when blended by a superior nose.

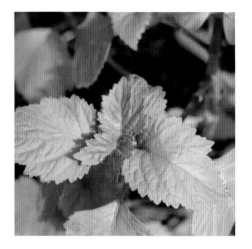

BLENDS WELL WITH
Citrus: bergamot
Floral: clary sage
Spicy: black pepper, cinnamon, clove
Woody: cedarwood

CAN BE SUBSTITUTED WITH
Oakmoss

PRECAUTIONS
May interact with certain medications. Talk to your doctor or pharmacist about potential interactions.

PROPERTIES

Antibacterial, Antidepressant, Antifungal, Anti-inflammatory, Antimicrobial, Antiseptic, Aphrodisiac, Astringent, Cell regeneration, Febrifuge, Insecticide

POTENTIAL USES

Ants, Athlete's foot, Chapped skin, Constipation, Digestive issues, Eczema, Fungal infections, Heartburn, Insect bites, Oily skin, Yeast infections/thrush

PEPPERMINT

Mentha piperita

SCENT: MINTY   **NOTE:** TOP   **COST:** $

The plant we know as peppermint is a natural hybrid, a cross between spearmint and watermint, a plant that grows in damp places across Europe, Asia, and northwest Africa. The ancient Romans planted peppermint between the stepping-stones leading to their houses so that guests would be welcomed by the scent as they approached. Peppermint is used to flavor both food and medicine and as a fragrance in cosmetics. Drunk as a tea, it aids digestion.

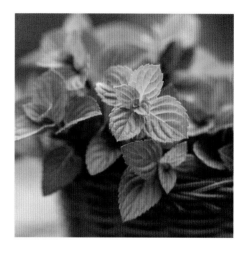

PROPERTIES
Analgesic, Antibacterial, Antiseptic, Decongestant, Febrifuge, Insecticide, Sedative, Vermifuge

POTENTIAL USES
Acne, Anxiety, Colds/flu, Congestion, Dermatitis, Digestive upset, Fever, Gas, Indigestion, Insect repellent, Itching, Motion sickness, Muscle aches, Nausea, Pest repellent, Ringworm, Vomiting, Scabies

BLENDS WELL WITH
Citrus: orange, lemon, grapefruilt
Floral: geranium
Medicinal: eucalyptus, tea tree, niaouli
Spicy: black pepper
Woody: benzoin

CAN BE SUBSTITUTED WITH
Spearmint

PRECAUTIONS
Avoid use while breastfeeding, as it can reduce the milk supply in some women.
Do not use with children under 6 years old.
Avoid use near mucous membranes.

PINE

Pinnus sylvestris

SCENT: WOODY   NOTE: MIDDLE   COST: $

Pine is an evergreen tree that can grow up to 115 feet high. The scent of pine oil is ubiquitous in cleaning products to the point that it is virtually synonymous with "clean." According to Bryan Miller and Dr. Light Miller, authors of the authoritative *Ayurveda & Aromatherapy*, "the world's largest production of any essential oil is pine." It is also used in perfumery in fragrances as diverse as Fille en Aiguilles by Serge Lutens and Black Forest by Black Phoenix Alchemy Lab.

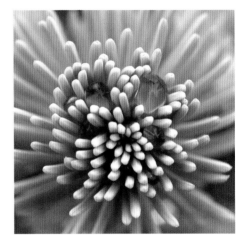

PROPERTIES
Analgesic, Antibacterial, Antidepressant, Antiseptic, Decongestant

POTENTIAL USES
Arthritis, Bronchitis, Cleaning products, Colds/flu, Congestion, Cough, Depression, Fatigue, Gout, Muscle aches, Scabies, Urinary tract infection

BLENDS WELL WITH
Citrus: bergamot, grapefruit, lemon, orange
Floral: lavender
Minty: peppermint
Medicinal: eucalyptus, tea tree
Oriental: frankincense
Woody: cedarwood

CAN BE SUBSTITUTED WITH
Cypress
Juniper

PRECAUTIONS
None specific.

ROSEMARY

Rosmarinus officinalis

SCENT: WOODY/HERBAL   **NOTE:** MIDDLE   COST: $

A cooking herb as well as an ingredient in many ancient medicines, rosemary is a perennial herb native to the Mediterranean. The scent has been known to stimulate memory since at least Shakespeare's time. ("There's rosemary; that's for remembrance," Ophelia says as she goes mad in *Hamlet*.) In Hoodoo folk magic traditions, rosemary is thought to empower women and is often used in spells to ward off evil. In astrology, rosemary is associated with Leo.

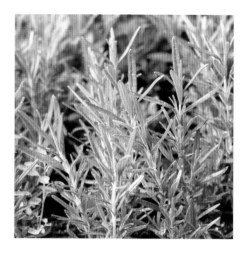

PROPERTIES

Antibacterial, Antifungal, Antiseptic, Astringent, Decongestant, Disinfectant, Expectorant, Stimulates hair growth, Stimulates memory

POTENTIAL USES

Aging skin, Athlete's foot, Bacterial infection, Cleaning products, Congestion, Cough, Dermatitis, Eczema, Gas, Hair loss, Heart palpitations, High blood pressure, Indigestion, Oily skin, Scabies

BLENDS WELL WITH

Citrus: lemon, lime, orange, grapefruit
Floral: lavender, clary sage
Herbal: basil
Medicinal: eucalyptus, tea tree
Minty: peppermint
Woody: pine

CAN BE SUBSTITUTED WITH

Basil
Thyme

PRECAUTIONS

Avoid use while pregnant.
Avoid use with children under 6 years old.

SANDALWOOD

Santalum album

SCENT: WOODY   **NOTE:** BOTTOM   **COST:** $$

Sandalwood is slightly more expensive than other woody essential oils, but its scent is highly prized. It has a woody, masculine scent found in incense, men's cologne, and women's fragrances. While traditional sandalwood comes from India, recently Australia has surpassed India as the leading provider of sandalwood throughout the world.

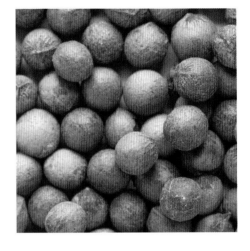

PROPERTIES
Anti-inflammatory, Antiseptic, Decongestant, Expectorant, Tonic

POTENTIAL USES
Acne, Dry skin, Colds/flu, Cough, Sinusitis, Urinary tract infection

BLENDS WELL WITH
Floral: petitgrain, rose, jasmine, ylang ylang
Woody: pine, benzoin

CAN BE SUBSTITUTED WITH
Cedarwood
Vetiver

PRECAUTIONS
None specific

TEA TREE

Melaleuca alternifolia

SCENT: MEDICINAL   **NOTE:** MIDDLE   **COST:** $

Tea tree oil is used to treat a variety of skin conditions, from acne to herpes. It has been shown to kill the superbug MRSA in a laboratory setting. In addition to its medicinal uses, tea tree has a long tradition of being used for energy work, aura cleansing, protection, purification, to open mental channels, and promote mental clarity. A native of Australia, the plant was named by British explorer Captain James Cook. It is associated with the moon and with Mercury.

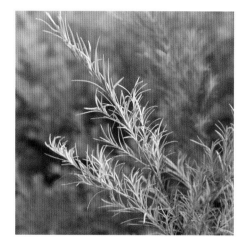

PROPERTIES
Antibacterial, Antifungal, Antiseptic, Antiviral, Cicatrizant, Expectorant, Febrifuge, Immune system stimulant, Insecticide

POTENTIAL USES
Abscesses, Acne, Athlete's foot, Bronchitis, Burns, Colds/flu, Corns, Cough, Dandruff, Fever, Fungal infections, Insect bites, Lice, Rash, Warts

BLENDS WELL WITH
Citrus: lemon, orange, lime
Floral: geranium, lavender
Herbal: basil
Minty: eucalyptus, peppermint
Spicy: black pepper, clove
Woody: pine

CAN BE SUBSTITUTED WITH
Cajeput
Lavender
Niaouli

PRECAUTIONS
None specific

VETIVER

Vetiveria zizanioide

SCENT: EARTHY   **NOTE:** BASE   COST: $$

Also known as "khus oil," vetiver is believed to be very calming and grounding. It is a perennial grass native to India that is often planted for erosion control. In folk magic it is said to be protective and it is used in rituals to attract money. The roots are used to make blinds, hats, and bags. The oil is extensively used in perfume where its earthy note is incorporated into fragrances like Encre Noire by Lalique, Vetiver by Zara, and Black Vetiver by Phaedon.

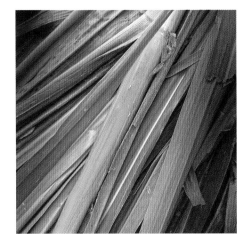

PROPERTIES
Antianxiety, Anti-inflammatory, Immune system booster, Scar healing, Sedative

POTENTIAL USES
Acne, Arthritis, Anxiety, Hyperactivity, Insomnia, Lowered immunity, Muscle aches/pains, Scarring, Stress

BLENDS WELL WITH
Citrus: orange, lemon, grapefruit, bergamot
Earthy: oakmoss, patchouli
Floral: rose, ylang ylang
Spicy: black pepper
Woody: sandalwood

CAN BE SUBSTITUTED WITH
Oakmoss
Patchouli

PRECAUTIONS
None specific.

YLANG YLANG

Cananga odorata

SCENT: FLORAL   **NOTE:** BASE   **COST:** $$

Known by many names, including "the perfume tree," ylang ylang is a fast-growing tree (up to 15 feet a year) native to the tropical rain forest in the Philippines and Malaysia. The plant is said to be an aphrodisiac and is used to treat nervous disorders and relieve stress. Ylang ylang oil is used extensively in perfumery. Some notable fragrances with ylang ylang notes are Ylang Austral by Givenchy and Ombre D'Or by Jean Charles Brosseau.

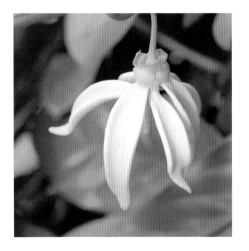

PROPERTIES
Aphrodisiac, Sedative, Tonic

POSSIBLE USES
Anxiety, Depression, Emotional trauma, Hair care, Skincare, Stress

BLENDS WELL WITH
Citrus: bergamot, orange
Earthy: vetiver
Floral: palmarosa, jasmine
Medicinal: eucalyptus
Oriental: patchouli
Woody: rosewood, sandalwood

CAN BE SUBSTITUTED WITH
Frangipani

PRECAUTIONS
Avoid use with children under 2 years old.
May irritate sensitive skin.

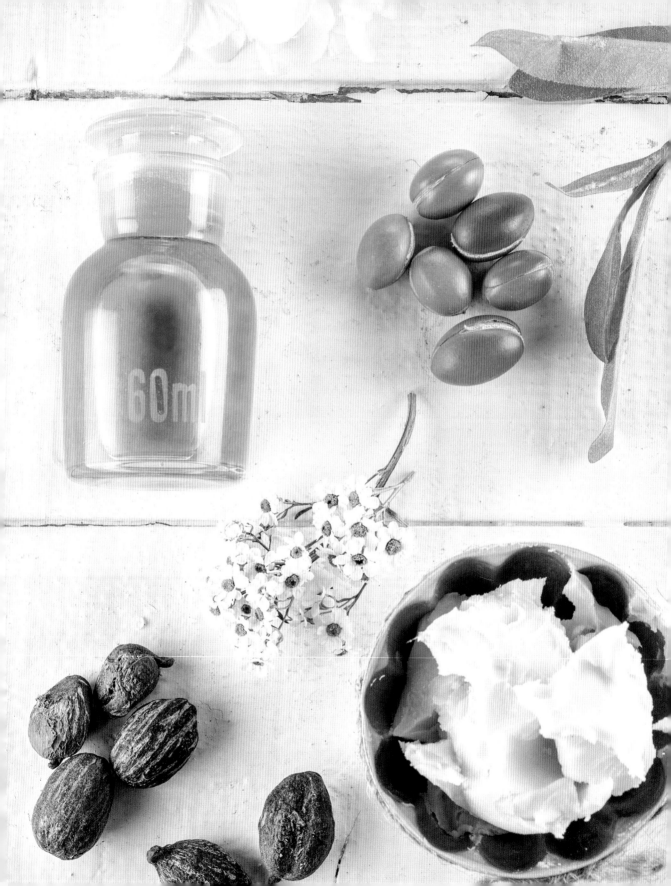

5

REMEDIES FOR HEALTH & HEALING

Anxiety 89 Arthritis 91 Athlete's Foot and Food Odor 93 Bad Breath 96

Bites and Stings 98 Blisters 101 Body Odor 103 Bruises 105 Burns 107

Colds, Coughs, and Congestion 109 Constipation 111 Cradle Cap 113

Cuts 115 Depression (mild) 117 Diaper rash 120 Digestive Problems 122

Ear Infection 124 Eczema and Rashes 126 Erectile Dysfunction 128

Flu 130 Headache 132 Hemorrhoids 134 Infection 136

Lice and Ringworm 138 Menopause 140 Morning Sickness 142

Muscle Aches 144 PMS 145 Seasonal Affective Disorder (SAD) 147

Sinus Pain 149 Sunburn 151 Toothache 153 Urinary Tract Infection (UTI) 154

Varicose Veins 156 Yeast Infection 158

Aromatherapy has been used for centuries to improve health and fight illness. Today, it serves as a complementary therapy to Western medicine. For minor ailments, many people choose to turn to natural solutions like aromatherapy at home, instead of using over-the-counter pharmaceutical products.

Aromatherapy remedies may include salves, lotions, massage oils, baths, and a host of other applications. These aromatherapy remedies may help reduce the toxic load placed on your body from over-the-counter medications, and they tend to be less expensive. However, if you are pregnant or breastfeeding or have a serious illness, talk to your primary health care provider about the use of aromatherapy, as it may be contraindicated with certain medications or conditions.

TAKE A DEEP BREATH CALMING DIFFUSION OIL

SCENT: MINT/CITRUS   COST: $

MAKES: 1 APPLICATION

This recipe is the peanut butter and jelly sandwich of aromatherapy. You can change it up by using lemon instead of orange, but the classic recipe is so calming that there's really no need to reinvent the wheel. The scent of orange brings about feelings of happiness, relaxation, and calm, while the scent of peppermint is believed to be calming and soothing.

DID YOU KNOW?

The ancients believed that orange oil was beneficial as a medicine for the spirit and the body because it was infused with solar energy.

2 drops peppermint essential oil
2 drops orange essential oil

Follow the directions for use of essential oils that come with your diffuser.

APPLICATION: While a diffuser or oil burner are your best choices, you can also add the essential oils to a hot bath, or to a bowl of steaming hot water to use them as a steam inhalant.

STORAGE: Use this diffusion blend immediately. You can also make up a larger batch and store it in a dark-colored glass bottle away from heat and light.

MASSAGE LOTION FOR BABIES

SCENT: FLORAL   COST: $$

MAKES: ½ CUP

A parent's touch can be all it takes to soothe a fretful baby, and giving your infant a gentle massage can also be soothing for you. The physical contact helps to develop the bond between a baby and parent, while massage can promote deep relaxation. Lavender (but only *Lavandula angustifolia*) is gentle enough to use with babies 3 months and older, while bergamot is safe for babies 6 months and older. For babies younger than 3 months, use just the apricot kernel oil, which is excellent for sensitive skin.

FOR BABIES 3 MONTHS AND OLDER

½ cup apricot kernel oil
2 drops lavender essential oil

FOR BABIES 6 MONTHS AND OLDER

½ cup apricot kernel oil
2 drops lavender essential oil
1 drop bergamot essential oil

In a 4-ounce bottle, combine the oil with the essential oil, and shake to blend.

APPLICATION: Shake before each use. Gently massage 1 teaspoon of oil onto the baby's skin or 1 tablespoon for an adult, replenishing as needed.

STORAGE: Store the bottle in a cool, dry spot for up to 12 months.

A CLOSER LOOK

Much of what is known about the importance of human touch for psychological well-being comes from a series of groundbreaking studies on the mother-infant bond conducted by Dr. Harry Harlow in the 1950s. His observations on what he called "contact comfort" and the dire results caused by maternal deprivation revolutionized the American approach to child-rearing, which had up to then been more hands-off so as not to "spoil children."

BASIC WARMING OIL

SCENT: SPICY   COST: $$

MAKES: ¼ CUP

This is a thermogenic essential oil blend, meaning it creates heat. The blend decreases pain and increases the flexibility of arthritic joints without the medicinal locker room smell of a commercial preparation like BenGay®. It's also far less expensive. The oil works on arthritic joints because it contains warming and analgesic oils such as cinnamon, nutmeg, black pepper, ginger, and clove along with anti-inflammatory oils such as sweet orange.

A CLOSER LOOK

There are more than 100 kinds of arthritis, but the most common is osteoarthritis, a degenerative joint disease that can be the result of trauma to the joint, infection of the joint, or aging. Although osteoarthritis can damage any joint in your body, the disorder most commonly affects joints in the hands, knees, hips, and spine.

2 ounces carrier oil
6 drops cinnamon essential oil
6 drops sweet orange essential oil
2 drops black pepper essential oil
2 drops nutmeg essential oil
2 drops ginger essential oil
2 drops clove essential oil

In a 2-ounce bottle, combine the carrier oil with the essential oils, and shake to blend.

APPLICATION: Shake the bottle before each use. Using 1 to 2 teaspoons, massage the warming oil blend gently into the inflamed joints once or twice a day, or as needed for pain.

STORAGE: Store the bottle in a cool, dry place for up to 12 months.

SMOTHERING THE FIRE OIL

SCENT: CITRUS/FLORAL   **COST:** $$

MAKES: 1 OUNCE

This soothing lotion contains essential oils that have anti-inflammatory properties to ease the pain in inflamed, stiff, swollen joints. The bergamot eases pain by numbing nerve endings, while the combined scent of bergamot and lavender lessens anxiety and the lemon promotes feelings of well-being. To avoid a buildup of specific essential oils in your system, alternate use of this lotion with the Basic Warming Oil on page 91.

1 ounce carrier oil

2 drops bergamot essential oil (or wild orange, which is cheaper)

2 drops lemon essential oil

2 drops lavender essential oil

In a 1-ounce bottle, combine the carrier oil with the essential oils and shake to blend.

APPLICATION: Shake the bottle before each use. Rub 1 or 2 teaspoons of the oil onto inflamed joints.

STORAGE: Store the tightly sealed bottle in a cool, dry place for up to 12 months.

TEA TREE AND LAVENDER FOOT POWDER

SCENT: MEDICINAL/FLORAL   COST: $

MAKES: 2 CUPS

If you've tried everything to treat your athlete's foot, including washing and bleaching your athletic shoes, sprinkling cornstarch into your socks, and wearing nothing but flip-flops, then you might want to try this synergistic blend of antifungal and astringent essential oils. This foot powder is also effective in treating foot odor. Cypress is a commonly used essential oil in deodorants because it's especially good at fighting odor. The addition of cosmetic clays, which are sold in powder form, helps absorb germs and toxins that may be contributing to odor and athlete's foot. If you suspect the foot odor is caused by athlete's foot, see a health care practitioner, as a serious bacterial infection may be present.

2 cups cosmetic clay
10 drops tea tree essential oil
5 drops lavender essential oil
5 drops cypress essential oil

1. In a ½-gallon plastic zip-top bag add the clay and then add the essential oils. Zip the bag closed and shake well to mix the ingredients.

2. Transfer the clay to a 16-ounce jar, preferably one with a shaker top.

APPLICATION: Sprinkle the powder onto the feet as needed, once or twice per day.

STORAGE: Tightly seal the shaker bottle and store in a cool, dry place for up to 12 months.

TIP
Shaker tops can be purchased online through General Bottle Supply (see Resources.)

PICKLE YOUR TOES FOOT BATH

SCENT: MEDICINAL   COST: $

MAKES: 1 TREATMENT

This foot soak combines the astringent qualities of apple cider vinegar and the serious antifungal action of tea tree oil to eliminate athlete's foot, fight odor, and soothe your feet. You don't need to find organic or unfiltered apple cider vinegar for this recipe. Any type will do. Save the more expensive apple cider vinegar for culinary uses—your feet won't mind.

TIP

Fungus breeds in dampness. Make sure to dry your feet thoroughly, using a hair dryer set on low to get between the toes.

1 gallon distilled water, warmed
5 cups apple cider vinegar
10 drops tea tree essential oil

1. In a foot tub or flat plastic tub, stir together the water and vinegar.

2. Add the tea tree oil, and stir to mix again.

APPLICATION: Soak your feet in the mixture for 10 to 20 minutes. When you're finished, you can use a cotton ball dipped in apple cider vinegar to dab onto itchy spots. Repeat the foot soak daily for 10 to 14 days.

STORAGE: This is a single-use treatment and should not be stored.

STINKY FEET SOAK

SCENT: HERBAL/FLORAL   COST: $$

MAKES: 1 TREATMENT

If you have chronically stinky feet, be sure to air them out as much as you can. When you are not at work, wear flip-flops instead of sneakers, which are breeding grounds for smells. Then, use this antimicrobial foot soak weekly to keep the odor-causing bacteria at bay. Baking soda is excellent for killing odor. Both vinegar and thyme kill bacteria and fungus that can contribute to odor, while lavender reduces body odor.

DID YOU KNOW?

Stress can make your feet smell bad.

4 cups warm water

4 cups white vinegar

½ cup baking soda

5 drops thyme essential oil

5 drops lavender essential oil

1. In a foot tub or flat plastic tub, combine the water and vinegar and mix well.

2. Add the baking soda and mix until it dissolves. (It may fizz a bit.)

3. Add the essential oils and agitate the water with your hands to mix it.

APPLICATION: Soak your feet in this blend once a week for at least 20 minutes. Dry your feet thoroughly after you are finished.

STORAGE: This is a single-use treatment and should not be stored.

BASIC MOUTHWASH

SCENT: SPICY   COST: $

MAKES: 1 CUP

Bad breath isn't always a sign of poor dental hygiene; it can also reveal the presence of an underlying medical condition such as diabetes or kidney disease. If bad breath is persistent or unusually foul, you may need to consult a doctor. This simple mouthwash cleanses and disinfects without drying out the tissues the way an alcohol-based mouth rinse can, which is beneficial as dry mouth may cause bad breath. The tea tree and clove essential oils also kill germs that may cause bad breath. Clove oil is commonly used in dental offices to dull nerve pain of toothaches, and this recipe may be helpful for the same purpose. If you prefer a different taste, feel free to substitute it with cinnamon, peppermint, or wintergreen essential oil.

1 cup water
15 drops clove essential oil
5 drops tea tree essential oil

In an 8-ounce bottle, combine the water with the essential oils, and shake well to blend.

APPLICATION: Shake before each use. Swish 1 to 2 tablespoons in your mouth and then spit out. Do not swallow the mouthwash.

STORAGE: Store the bottle in a cool, dark place for up to 12 months.

DID YOU KNOW?
According to Dr. Li Zhisui, private physician to Mao Zedong from 1954 to 1976, the Chinese leader never brushed his teeth, preferring to simply rinse his mouth with green tea instead.

MINTY MINERALIZING TOOTHPASTE

SCENT: MINTY   COST: $

MAKES: 2/3 CUP

Up until the middle of the 19th century, toothpaste as it is known today didn't exist. Many people have concerns about today's toothpaste because it contains a number of chemicals. This version is mild and nontoxic, but you still shouldn't swallow it. The calcium carbonate and baking soda provide a gentle abrasion, while the coconut oil and the tea tree and peppermint essential oils kill germs and freshen your breath.

TIP
If the paste is too bitter for your taste, add xylitol powder, a sweetener derived from birch trees, but also created chemically (see Resources).

5 tablespoons calcium carbonate
2 tablespoons baking soda
5 tablespoons extra-virgin coconut oil
12 drops peppermint essential oil
6 drops tea tree essential oil

1. In a small glass or metal bowl, mix together the calcium carbonate and baking soda.

2. Stir in the coconut oil 1 tablespoon at a time until the paste reaches the desired consistency.

3. Add the essential oils, mixing well. Then transfer the mixture to a 6-ounce bottle.

APPLICATION: Put a small amount of toothpaste on a toothbrush and brush your teeth.

STORAGE: Store the tightly sealed bottle in a cool, dry place for up to 12 months.

ANTIBACTERIAL SOAP WITH ROSEMARY AND THYME

SCENT: HERBACEOUS/MINTY   COST: $$

MAKES: 1 CUP

In case of an animal bite, it's important to clean the site very thoroughly before applying any first aid treatment. Wash with this antibiotic soap and hot water to remove any bacteria that may have come from the animal's mouth. For severe bites, or if you are concerned about rabies, seek immediate medical attention. This antibiotic soap is also fine to use for regular hand-washing.

TIP

For this recipe, you'll need a foaming-soap dispenser, which is designed to convert the soap to a creamy foam as you use it. You can either repurpose a bottle you have or buy one new (see Resources).

⅔ cup water

2 tablespoons unscented liquid castile soap

2 teaspoons carrier oil

10 drops rosemary essential oil

10 drops tea tree essential oil

5 drops thyme essential oil

5 drops peppermint essential oil

5 drops cinnamon essential oil

4 drops eucalyptus essential oil

1. In a 1-quart glass measuring cup, vigorously mix together the water, soap, and carrier oil.

2. Add the essential oils and mix well.

3. Using a funnel, transfer the mixture to an 8-ounce foam-soap dispenser bottle.

APPLICATION: Use this soap as needed or for general washing of hands, using 1 pump of the soap from the dispenser per use.

STORAGE: Store the foam dispenser at room temperature. This soap should last for 3 to 6 months.

THE EASIEST MOSQUITO BITE REMEDY EVER

SCENT: FLORAL   COST: $

MAKES: 1 OUNCE

If you didn't apply your bug repellent soon enough, and you now have one (or ten) mosquito bites, this is a one-drop stop for mosquito bite itching and pain. The lavender oil is soothing, relaxing, and calming, and should remove the itch from the bite.

2 teaspoons carrier oil

4 teaspoons lavender essential oil

1. In a small glass or metal bowl, mix the carrier oil and the lavender essential oil.

2. Pour the oil into a roller bottle before applying to the bite.

SIMPLE SWAP

Other essential oils can be used to remove the itch, as well. These include chamomile, lemon, tea tree oil, and niaouli essential oils.

APPLICATION: Roll the mixture onto the bites to stop the itching.

STORAGE: Store in the tightly sealed roller bottle in a cool, dark place for up to 12 months.

ANTI-STING BEE STING PASTE

SCENT: FLORAL   COST: $

MAKES: 1 TREATMENT

Bee stings can be very uncomfortable, first stinging and then itching. This healing paste uses baking soda to immediately remove the sting and absorb the venom and includes lavender essential oil to soothe and calm inflammation. Flick the stinger away from the skin immediately to prevent more venom from pumping into the wound, and then carefully dab the paste on the sting. If you are allergic to bee stings, seek immediate medical attention.

DID YOU KNOW?

Throughout history bee venom has been used to treat pain in much the same way that capsicum-based pepper creams are used today. Greek physician Hippocrates used bee venom to treat arthritis more than two thousand years ago.

1 teaspoon baking soda
2 drops lavender essential oil
A few drops of distilled water

1. In a small glass bowl, mix together the baking soda and lavender essential oil.

2. Add just enough water, working in a few drops at a time, to form a paste.

APPLICATION: Dab the paste over the sting after removing the stinger.

STORAGE: This is a single-use treatment and does not require storage.

GERANIUM–CALENDULA BLISTER GEL

SCENT: FLORAL   COST: $

MAKES: 1 OUNCE

Perhaps one of the worst and best things about blisters is that you can feel them forming. If you can't stop whatever you are doing to avoid developing the blister in the first place, this gel can help to heal the skin and dull the pain. The geranium oil is an astringent and shrinks tissue. The calendula helps fight inflammation, while the aloe vera gel soothes and cools. Together they may help ease the pain of blisters.

1 ounce pure aloe vera gel
5 drops calendula essential oil
1 drop geranium essential oil

In a 1-ounce bottle, combine the aloe vera gel and the essential oils and mix using a metal rod.

APPLICATION: Dab a small amount of the gel on the blister and cover it with a bandage, once or twice per day.

STORAGE: Store the tightly sealed bottle in a cool, dry place for up to 12 months.

DID YOU KNOW?
You should never pop a blister. Gently wash it with soap and water and cover it with gel and a bandage. Popping a blister can be painful and may lead to infection.

FREEZE-OUT FEVER BLISTER OINTMENT

SCENT: MEDICINAL/MINTY   COST: $

MAKES: 1 OUNCE

A virus causes fever blisters, which can be very painful. If you've had even one, there is a chance they will recur. You can use this ointment to both prevent fever blisters and to treat them. It contains tea tree and peppermint essential oils, which have antiviral properties. If you already have a fever blister (aka a cold sore), dab the ointment directly on the sore using a clean cotton swab. If you think one is about to form, spread a little on the area and let it go to work.

1 ounce carrier oil
5 drops tea tree essential oil
1 drop peppermint essential oil

In a 1-ounce bottle, combine the carrier oil with the essential oils and shake to blend.

APPLICATION: Shake before each use. With a clean cotton swab, dab a little of the ointment on the affected area once or twice per day.

STORAGE: Store the bottle in a cool, dry place for up to 12 months.

DID YOU KNOW?

Fever blisters, also known as cold sores, are a form of herpes. They appear on the mouth and face, but the virus can be transmitted to the genitals. They are highly contagious. About 90 percent of Americans have had at least one cold sore, and 40 percent have repeated cold sores. They can be triggered by stress, the onset of a menstrual period, a dental procedure, or even exposure to the sun or wind.

TEA TREE & LEMON DEODORANT

SCENT: MEDICINAL/CITRUS   COST: $

MAKES: 1 DEODORANT STICK

This deodorant is not only quick and easy to make but also does not contain aluminum, which some evidence has linked to Alzheimer's disease. The shea butter and cocoa butter are highly moisturizing, which keeps your armpits well conditioned. The cornstarch absorbs moisture to prevent odor, while the tea tree and lemon essential oils fight odor-causing bacteria. If you don't have an empty stick deodorant container handy, you can buy them new on Amazon.

SIMPLE SWAP

Don't enjoy the medicinal scent of the tea tree essential oil? Try replacing it with geranium essential oil, instead, which has a more floral, less medicinal scent.

2 tablespoons shea butter
1 tablespoon cocoa butter
2 tablespoons cornstarch
1 tablespoon baking soda
2 teaspoons aloe vera gel
10 drops tea tree essential oil
10 drops lemon essential oil

1. Fill a medium saucepan with a few inches of water and set it on the stove over low heat. Place a metal or glass bowl over the pan so that it fits well.

2. Add the shea and cocoa butters to the bowl and stir as they melt. (You can also nuke them in the microwave, which will take about 2 minutes. Stop and stir after each 20-second burst).

3. Stir in the remaining ingredients and mix until the cornstarch and baking soda have dissolved.

4. Transfer the mixture into an empty deodorant container and put it into the refrigerator to harden.

APPLICATION: Apply as you would commercially bought deodorant to underarms once a day.

STORAGE: Store the capped deodorant container in a cool, dry place for up to 12 months.

TEA TREE AND JUNIPER BODY WASH

SCENT: MEDICINAL/WOODY   COST: $

MAKES: ½ CUP

This is an easy recipe to make. Castile soap is a pure vegetable-based soap and has a number of uses beyond a body wash. This recipe uses antibacterial tea tree essential oil to fight odor-causing germs, and juniper to remove body toxins that may cause odor. The vitamin E capsule serves multiple functions, working as an antioxidant and skin moisturizer, as well as a preservative to keep the body wash fresh longer. Both of the essential oils used here are invigorating, making this body wash a great way to start out the day.

SIMPLE SWAP

Juniper oil has a woody scent that tends to be very masculine. For a brighter scent, replace the juniper with orange, bergamot, or grapefruit oil.

½ cup liquid pure castile soap
1 tablespoon carrier oil
3 vitamin E capsules
25 drops tea tree essential oil
25 drops juniper essential oil

1. In a dark-colored, 8-ounce bottle, combine the soap and the carrier oil, and shake vigorously to mix well.

2. Pierce the vitamin E capsules and squeeze the oil into the soap mixture.

3. Add the essential oils, and shake well to blend.

APPLICATION: Shake well before each use. Use 1 to 2 tablespoons of soap daily in the shower or bath.

STORAGE: Keep the wash stored in the tightly sealed bottle for up to 12 months. If you are concerned about having a glass bottle in your bath or shower, a dark-colored plastic bottle can be used instead as long as the wash isn't stored in the bottle for long periods.

COMFREY BRUISE HEALING OIL

SCENT: HERBAL   COST: $

MAKES: 1 OUNCE

Comfrey isn't an essential oil, but rather an oil made via herbal infusion. You can find it in many health food stores. Comfrey is well known for its bruise healing properties, primarily from a chemical it contains called allantoin, which is anti-inflammatory. Helichrysum essential oil serves as an anti-inflammatory oil that helps to reduce pain and swelling.

1 ounce carrier oil
6 drops comfrey herbal oil
3 drops helichrysum essential oil

In a 1-ounce bottle, combine the carrier oil, Comfrey, and essential oil and shake to blend.

APPLICATION: Shake before using. Gently massage about 1 teaspoon of the oil on the affected area.

STORAGE: Store the tightly sealed bottle in a cool, dry place for up to 12 months.

SIMPLE SWAP

If you can't find comfrey oil or you don't have any on hand, it can be replaced with an equal amount of lavender, rosemary, or calendula essential oils.

ROSEMARY-LAVENDER SALVE FOR BRUISES

SCENT: HERBAL/FLORAL   COST: $$

MAKES: 1½ CUPS

Use this salve in conjunction with ice for severe bruises to help decrease inflammation. Both rosemary and lavender have anti-inflammatory properties that can shrink swelling of bruises and remove the pain.

½ cup beeswax
1 cup carrier oil
1 vitamin E capsule
24 drops lavender essential oil
24 drops rosemary essential oil

1. Fill a small saucepan with a few inches of water and set it on the stove over low heat. Place a metal or glass bowl over the pan so that it fits well.

2. Add the beeswax to the bowl and wait until it melts. Then stir in the carrier oil.

3. Pierce the vitamin E capsule and squeeze the vitamin E oil into the beeswax mix.

4. Add the lavender and rosemary essential oils and mix well.

5. Transfer to a 12-ounce jar, and allow it to cool before putting on the lid.

APPLICATION: Dab a small amount of the salve onto the bruised area using a light touch. Reapply 2 to 3 times daily until swelling and pain diminish.

STORAGE: Store the tightly sealed jar in a cool, dry place for up to 12 months.

BASIC BURN GEL

SCENT: MEDICINAL COST: $

MAKES: 1 OUNCE

A first-degree burn—like the kind you get from touching a hot pan—is easy to treat by running the affected area under cold water and patting it dry. A second-degree burn involves blisters and more layers of damaged skin, and needs to be treated with more care. If there are any signs of infection or if the burn is more serious than a bad sunburn, seek medical help immediately. For minor burns, use this cooling aloe vera–based gel to soothe the pain.

SIMPLE SWAP

To make this gel for children, replace the helichrysum essential oil with 6 drops each of rosemary and lavender essential oils.

1 ounce pure aloe vera gel
12 drops helichrysum essential oil

In a 1-ounce bottle, combine the gel and the essential oil and mix using a metal spoon.

APPLICATION: Dab a small amount on the affected area and cover it loosely with gauze.

STORAGE: Store the tightly sealed jar in a cool, dry spot for up to 12 months.

NUMBING SUNBURN SPRAY

SCENT: MEDICINAL   COST: $

MAKES: 1 CUP

There are a lot of anesthetizing and numbing pain-relief sprays on the market. Many contain the numbing medication lidocaine, which provides temporary pain relief. These sprays don't smell very good, and they can be expensive. However, many essential oils have analgesic properties to reduce pain associated with burns. Before you resort to one of the over-the-counter remedies, try this soothing analgesic, anti-inflammatory spray with cooling peppermint essential oil.

1 cup distilled water
15 drops lavender essential oil
15 drops peppermint essential oil
10 drops rosemary essential oil

In an 8-ounce spray bottle, combine the water and the essential oils and shake to mix well.

APPLICATION: Shake before using. Spray a small amount on the affected area 2 to 3 times per day. Cover the area loosely with gauze.

STORAGE: Store the spray bottle in a cool, dry location for up to 12 months.

EUCALYPTUS–MINT RUB

SCENT: MEDICINAL/MINT   **COST:** $

MAKES: 1 OUNCE

Scent is well known for its effectiveness at relieving congestion, which is the principle behind the Vicks VapoRub your mom used to rub on your chest when you had a cold. This affordable and natural home remedy contains only natural coconut oil and essential oils. Almost any of the minty, medicinal, camphor-like scents can be used in this decongestant rub in place of the eucalyptus or peppermint. For a similarly effective hot bath, put 3 drops each of eucalyptus and peppermint essential oil into the bath and soak for 15 minutes, breathing deeply.

1 ounce extra-virgin coconut oil
6 drops eucalyptus essential oil
6 drops peppermint essential oil

1. Fill a bowl halfway full with hot water and set a 1-ounce jar with the lid removed in the bowl so the water goes about halfway up the side of the jar.

2. Add the coconut oil to the jar and allow it to melt.

3. Stir in the essential oils.

4. Remove the jar from the water bath and dry the sides. Screw the lid on the jar.

APPLICATION: Rub 1 teaspoon of the salve on the chest twice a day to relieve congestion.

STORAGE: Store the tightly sealed container in a cool, dry place for up to 12 months.

WARNING

Do not use eucalyptus essential oil with children under 10 years old. You can replace it with cypress, fir, pine, spruce, or juniper essential oils. In general, peppermint essential oil should not be used with children 6 years old or younger.

ROSEMARY–LEMON–EUCALYPTUS RUB

SCENT: MEDICINAL/CITRUS   COST: $

MAKES: APPROXIMATELY ¾ CUP

This combination of scents is one of the go-to combos for an essential oil treatment of colds. Both eucalyptus and rosemary essential oils have decongestant properties, while lemon oil strengthens immunity and helps fight infection. All the ingredients fight bacteria and contain antidepressive properties to help boost your mood.

DID YOU KNOW?
The Smith Brothers were the original creators of cough drops, and they made them with menthol, which cooled the cough and eased congestion.

1 tablespoon grated beeswax
7 tablespoons extra-virgin coconut oil
20 drops rosemary essential oil
20 drops eucalyptus essential oil
20 drops lemon essential oil

1. Fill a small saucepan with a few inches of water and set it on the stove over low heat. Place a metal or glass bowl over the pan so that it fits well.

2. Add the beeswax to the bowl and wait until it melts. Then stir in the coconut oil until it is melted.

3. Remove the bowl from the heat and add the essential oils, mixing well.

4. Transfer the mixture to a 6-ounce glass jar, and allow it to cool before putting on the lid.

APPLICATION: Rub about 1 teaspoon of this salve on the chest to relieve congestion once or twice a day.

STORAGE: Store the tightly sealed container in a cool, dry location for up to 12 months.

UNCLENCH MASSAGE BLEND

SCENT: MINTY/SPICY   COST: $

MAKES: 1 OUNCE

Peppermint's purpose in life seems to be in aiding human digestion. Whether taken internally as a tea or rubbed on with a massage, the essential oil's antispasmodic and calmative properties help the muscles in the sphincter relax, which may ease constipation. The black pepper oil is warming, and it is also an antispasmodic, which can relax intestinal walls to help get things moving.

SIMPLE SWAP
If you don't have black pepper essential oil, try substituting ginger or rosemary oil instead.

1 ounce carrier oil
4 drops peppermint essential oil
2 drops black pepper essential oil

In a 1-ounce bottle, combine all the ingredients, and shake to blend well.

APPLICATION: Shake before each use. Rub 1 teaspoon of the oil onto the abdomen using light, clockwise circular strokes as needed, once or twice a day.

STORAGE: Store the tightly sealed bottle in a cool, dark place for up to 12 months.

DIGESTION BATH

SCENT: MINTY/ORANGE   **COST:** $

MAKES: 1 TREATMENT

Peppermint essential oil—even just a couple of drops of it—is antispasmodic, aids the digestion, and soothes the stomach while orange essential oil acts as a tonic and digestive. When combined in a hot bath, this blend may aid digestion, soothe an upset stomach, and increase relaxation. While in the bath, rub your abdomen in a circular motion, clockwise, with the flat of your hand two or three times to further relax bowels.

DID YOU KNOW?

This bath mixture can also serve as an effective and wonderfully fragrant exfoliator. Try doubling the recipe and using just half of it in the bath. After drying off, use your fingers to rub some of the mixture onto the bottom of your feet. Rub around the heels and ankles until the oil is absorbed, and then put on socks.

1 ounce Epsom salts
1 tablespoon carrier oil
3 drops sweet orange essential oil
2 drops peppermint essential oil

1. In a small bowl, add the Epsom salts and then the carrier oil. Mix well.

2. Add the sweet orange and peppermint essential oils to the bowl, and mix again.

3. Run a warm bath and then add the salt and essential oils mixture to it, agitating the water with your hands to fully incorporate it.

APPLICATION: Soak in the warm bath for about 15 minutes.

STORAGE: This is a single-use treatment, so no storage is necessary.

ESSENTIAL CRADLE CAP OIL BLEND

SCENT: FLORAL/CITRUS/WOODY **COST:** $$

MAKES: 1 OUNCE

With any essential oil treatment intended for infants and babies, be particularly cautious in diluting the oils. You can treat cradle cap by gently rubbing a little warmed olive oil over the affected area, but these gentle remedies will help soothe the skin and hasten the healing. Cradle cap, which often appears as scaly crusts on the scalp, is a medical condition also known as infantile seborrheic dermatitis and is very common in babies. Do not use on babies under 6 months old.

1 ounce sweet almond oil
1 drop lemon essential oil
1 drop geranium essential oil
1 drop cedarwood essential oil
1 drop sandalwood essential oil

In a 1-ounce bottle, mix the almond oil with the essential oils, and shake to blend.

APPLICATION: Shake before each use. Gently rub about a ¼ to a ½ teaspoon of oil on the affected area once a day.

STORAGE: Store the tightly sealed bottle in a cool, dark place for up to 12 months.

SIMPLE SWAP

Sandalwood essential oil is moderately expensive (between $15 and $20 per 5 mL) and can be substituted with a second drop of cedarwood essential oil.

GENTLE LAVENDER OIL BLEND

SCENT: FLORAL   COST: $

MAKES: 1 OUNCE

This remedy is safe for babies 3 months and older because lavender is very gentle. Use a gentle carrier oil, such as apricot kernel or sweet almond oil to further help with cradle cap. In addition to its disinfectant and skin-soothing properties, lavender is also a relaxant and soporific, which may help soothe a fretful baby. Don't use this more than once per day for five days. Take a break for at least two days before applying the blend again.

1 ounce carrier oil
4 drops lavender essential oil

In a 1-ounce bottle, combine the carrier oil and the essential oil, and shake to blend.

APPLICATION: Shake before each use. Gently massage ¼ to ½ teaspoon of oil onto your baby's scalp once a day for up to 5 days.

STORAGE: Store the tightly sealed bottle in a cool, dry location for up to 12 months.

TEA TREE OIL TREATMENT

SCENT: MEDICINAL   COST: $

MAKES: 1 TREATMENT

Cuts, whether the annoying slice of a paper cut or a kitchen accident, are a fact of life. Tea tree essential oil is a strong antiseptic, and one of the few oils that can be applied without dilution. Here it is paired with another powerful germ-fighter, rosemary essential oil, to powerfully protect against bacteria. Clean the wound first with the Antibacterial Soap with Rosemary and Thyme (page 98) before applying the treatment.

1 teaspoon carrier oil
1 drop tea tree essential oil
1 drop rosemary essential oil

Pour the ingredients into the palm of your clean hand and mix with a finger.

APPLICATION: This treatment is for use on small cuts only. Using a clean, dry cotton swab, apply a small dab of the oil directly on the cut once or twice a day. Cover cut with a bandage.

STORAGE: This is a single-use treatment, so no storage is required.

DID YOU KNOW?
If you have a cut finger, stick it in a small amount of plain white flour. The blood and the flour will form a glue that will seal the cut and stop the bleeding. Brush off the excess flour and cover with an adhesive bandage to protect the wound. Discard the remaining flour.

TEA TREE GEL

SCENT: MEDICINAL   COST: $

MAKES: 1 OUNCE

The tea tree essential oil in this gel keeps bacteria away, while the aloe vera gel soothes and reduces inflammation associated with cuts. Be sure to carefully clean the cut before applying the gel, and then cover it with a bandage to keep out bacteria and allow the wound to heal.

1 ounce pure aloe vera gel

6 drops tea tree essential oil

In a 1-ounce bottle, combine the aloe vera with the tea tree essential oil. Mix them together with a metal spoon.

APPLICATION: Dab a small amount of the gel on the affected area using a clean cotton swab and cover it with a bandage.

STORAGE: Store the tightly sealed glass bottle in a cool, dry place for up to 12 months.

HAPPINESS IS A WARM BATH

SCENT: CITRUS/HERBAL   COST: $

MAKES: 1 CUP

There are no quick fixes when it comes to depression, which makes it difficult to do or find pleasure in much of anything. But a warm bath can bring a much-needed moment of relaxation and release from the prison that even mild depression can feel like. This is a soothing soak that's infused with a blend of essential oils designed to quiet anxiety and lift mood. This combination of grapefruit and juniper is a favorite spa blend for detoxification and relaxation.

TIP

Sometimes depression can be brought on by an intensely stressful situation. But if you're also experiencing feelings of helplessness or hopelessness, and a general apathy, it might be time to seek out a health care professional. For more information consult Help Guide, a clearinghouse of resources on mental health: www.helpguide.org.

½ cup sea salt
½ cup baking soda
3 drops grapefruit essential oil
3 drops juniper essential oil

1. In a metal or glass bowl, combine the salt and the baking soda.

2. Add the grapefruit and juniper essential oils and mix until there aren't any clumps in the salt.

3. Store in a small mason jar or other airtight container.

APPLICATION: Add a ¼ cup of bath salts to running bathwater. Soak for 15 minutes once a day.

STORAGE: Store, tightly sealed, in a small container in a cool, dry location for up to 12 months.

FIVE FLOWER BALM

SCENT: FLORAL   COST: $$

MAKES: 2 OUNCES

Technically, this is a blend of three flowers, a wood, and a fruit, which sounds like the title of an indie movie. The balm is luxurious and nourishing, and the addition of a few drops of evening primrose oil gives it a little extra boost in lifting mood, particularly when combined with warm sandalwood essential oil and feel-good geranium essential oil.

A CLOSER LOOK

When you are using carrier oil, it usually doesn't matter which type you use. But once you start using substances that are solid at room temperature, such as coconut oil, shea butter, or cocoa butter, it gets a little trickier. Cocoa butter is hard at room temperature while shea butter is soft. If you switch them in recipes, the end product might not turn out the way you'd hoped.

1 tablespoon beeswax
¼ cup almond oil
5 drops evening primrose oil
5 drops palmarosa essential oil
5 drops geranium essential oil
5 drops lemon essential oil
5 drops sandalwood essential oil

1. Fill a small saucepan with a few inches of water and set it on the stove over low heat. Place a metal or glass bowl over the pan so that it fits well.

2. Add the beeswax to the bowl and wait until it melts. Then pour in the almond oil and add the drops of evening primrose oil.

3. Remove the bowl from the heat and add the rest of the essential oils.

4. Transfer the mixture to a 5-ounce glass or ceramic bottle with a pump top and allow it to cool completely before putting on the top.

APPLICATION: Apply a few tablespoons of the lotion once or twice a day as needed.

STORAGE: Store the bottle in a cool, dry location for up to 12 months.

DE-STRESS BATH SALTS

SCENT: WOODY/SPICY   COST: $–$$

MAKES: 2 CUPS

Epsom salts are made from magnesium sulfate. Magnesium is a mineral that promotes relaxation, which makes it a great addition to a calming bath. Meanwhile, patchouli and lavender oils both have antidepressant properties. The fir needle oil adds a pleasant woody scent that allows you to relax.

1 cup sea salt

1 cup Epsom salts

20 drops patchouli essential oil

15 drops fir needle essential oil (or pine or spruce)

15 drops lavender essential oil

1. In a 16-ounce glass or ceramic jar, combine the sea salt and Epsom salts, and mix well.

2. Sprinkle the essential oils evenly over the salts and stir.

GIFT IT

Customized bath salts are the ultimate DIY gift. You can present them in simple mason jars or those ubiquitous square jars. Add a label and a little scoop, along with a plush washcloth or hand towel, and you have a luxury spa gift.

APPLICATION: Use about a ¼ cup of the salts in a warm bath as needed.

STORAGE: Store the tightly sealed jar in a cool, dark location for up to 12 months.

CHAMOMILE–CALENDULA DIAPER CREAM

SCENT: FLORAL   COST: $$

MAKES: APPROXIMATELY 1 CUP

Chamomile essential oil is slightly more expensive than some other essential oils, but it isn't off-the-charts expensive and a little of this gentle oil goes a very long way. Therefore, it's well worth the cost of a small bottle so you have it available for multiple uses. Using just a few drops at a time keeps it relatively affordable, and it's such an outstanding ingredient, it's well worth the price. Cornstarch makes a good substitute for arrowroot powder, and lavender essential oil can be used in place of the chamomile.

TIP

There are many different types of chamomile oil, such as Roman, German, and blue chamomile oil. They all work interchangeably, so find the chamomile essential oil that best meets your budgetary needs.

½ cup shea butter
½ cup extra-virgin coconut oil
1 teaspoon arrowroot powder
1 teaspoon calendula oil
8 drops chamomile essential oil

1. Fill a small saucepan with a few inches of water and set it on the stove over low heat. Place a metal or glass bowl over the pan so that it fits well.

2. Add the shea butter and the coconut oil to the bowl, stirring as they melt.

3. Remove the bowl from the heat and stir in the arrowroot powder.

4. Stir in the calendula and chamomile essential oils using a metal spoon or glass stirring rod.

5. Transfer the mixture to an 8-ounce, wide-mouth jar, and allow it to cool and harden before putting on the lid.

APPLICATION: Apply a ¼ to a ½ teaspoon of the balm to the affected area once or twice per day.

STORAGE: Store the tightly sealed jar in a cool, dark place for up to 12 months.

BABY BUM LOTION

SCENT: FLORAL   COST: $$

MAKES: APPROXIMATELY 1 CUP

This healing lotion can be used with a soft baby washcloth. Castile soap is gentle, while the carrier oil and vitamin E add soothing moisture. The vitamin E also serves as a baby-safe preservative that's a lot more natural than the ingredients in commercially available diaper wipes or rash treatments. The lavender and chamomile gently soothe baby's rash. This lotion can be used on babies 6 months and older.

DID YOU KNOW?

Cloth diapers were first mass-produced in the United States in 1887 by an entrepreneur named Maria Allen.

1 tablespoon carrier oil
1 tablespoon unscented liquid castile soap
1 cup distilled water
1 vitamin E capsule
3 drops lavender essential oil
2 drops chamomile essential oil

1. In a small bowl, combine the carrier oil, soap, and water and mix well.

2. Pierce the vitamin E capsule and squeeze the oil out into the mixture.

3. Add the essential oils and stir. Pour into a 10-ounce spray bottle.

APPLICATION: Shake well before each use. Spray 1 or 2 spritzes on your baby's bottom once or twice a day. Rub in gently.

STORAGE: Store the tightly sealed spray bottle in a cool, dark location for up to 12 months.

GAS RELIEF RUB

SCENT: MINTY/HERBAL   COST: $

MAKES: 1 TREATMENT

Gas can be very uncomfortable, both socially and physically. Rubbing this essential oil–infused massage oil over the stomach can help soothe and dissipate gas that builds up in the intestinal tract. Fennel is an excellent stomach soother—both ingested as an herb and used topically in essential oil. Peppermint is also well tested as a gas reliever.

¼ cup carrier oil

3 drops peppermint essential oil

3 drops fennel essential oil

In a small glass or metal bowl, combine the carrier oil and the essential oils, and mix well.

APPLICATION: Using the flat of your hands, gently massage the stomach in clockwise circles until the oil is absorbed.

STORAGE: This is a single-use treatment, so no storage is required.

DID YOU KNOW?

Long before the invention of chewable antacids (in the 1920s), licorice root was chewed to stop heartburn.

HERBAL INDIGESTION MASSAGE

SCENT: HERBAL   COST: $

MAKES: 1 TREATMENT

Many antacids today have mint flavoring, but the pleasant herbal aromas of thyme, rosemary, and marjoram essential oils make a nice change of pace. However, don't take these oils internally; instead, massage them gently on your belly in light circles, breathing deeply as you do. All have antispasmodic properties that can help ease indigestion.

DID YOU KNOW?

Overeating can cause heartburn because it puts a lot of pressure on the lower esophageal sphincter (LES), the valve between the esophagus and stomach. When you overeat, the pressure on that valve intensifies and stomach acid can belch up, leaving the upper digestive tract inflamed.

1 teaspoon carrier oil
2 drops thyme essential oil
1 drop marjoram essential oil
1 drop rosemary essential oil

In the palm of your hand, mix together the carrier oil and the essential oils.

APPLICATION: Gently massage onto the belly with the flat of the hand, moving clockwise in slow circles.

STORAGE: This is a single-use application and does not require storage.

TEA TREE OIL TREATMENT

SCENT: MEDICINAL   COST: $

MAKES: 2 OUNCES

This preparation uses two ingredients that have long been used as folk remedies for curing earaches. Olive oil helps to dissolve earwax buildup that may be contributing to pain, while tea tree essential oil has antibacterial and antiseptic properties that may help with any infection contributing to pain.

DID YOU KNOW?

Garlic oil has also been used to treat ear infections. A blend of mullein oil and garlic is commercially available from several essential oil suppliers.

¼ cup olive oil

12 to 24 drops tea tree essential oil

In a 2-ounce bottle with a dropper top, combine the olive oil with the tea tree essential oil, and shake to blend.

APPLICATION: Shake before each use. Put 6 drops of oil on a cotton ball and place it in the ear at the entrance to the ear canal. Leave it there for at least 15 minutes, and then discard the cotton ball.

STORAGE: Store the tightly sealed bottle in a cool, dry place for up to 12 months.

SWIMMER'S EAR RELIEF

SCENT: MEDICINAL   COST: $

MAKES: 1 TREATMENT

Swimmer's ear occurs when water gets too deep inside the ear canal to drain out, causing an infection. You should never put drops of essential oil directly in the ear canal unless directed to do so by a qualified professional practitioner. Instead, soaking a cotton ball and putting it in the outer ear at the base of the ear canal may help. Try healing basil essential oil, which is tonic and antiseptic and also serves to draw mucus to the surface.

1 teaspoon carrier oil
1 drop basil essential oil

In a small glass or metal bowl, mix the carrier oil and essential oil.

APPLICATION: Soak a cotton ball in the mixture, then place the cotton ball in the ear at the base of the ear canal. Leave it there for at least 15 minutes, and then discard the cotton ball.

STORAGE: This is a single-dose application and does not require storage.

BABY-SAFE SALVE

SCENT: FLORAL/HERBAL/MEDICINAL   COST: $

MAKES: 4 TO 6 APPLICATIONS

"Rash" is a catchall term that includes the itchy inflammation and discoloration caused by a variety of conditions ranging from poison ivy and dermatitis to hives and heat rash. Eczema, impetigo, and psoriasis are just three of the many different kinds of rashes. The important thing in treating a rash is not to irritate the skin any more than it already is. This soothing, anti-itch formula is not just baby-safe, but it can also be used on dogs.

SIMPLE SWAP
For a slightly less medicinal scent, substitute niaouli essential oil for tea tree essential oil.

½ cup cocoa butter
¼ cup extra-virgin coconut oil
3 vitamin E capsules
20 drops geranium essential oil
15 drops lavender essential oil
15 drops cedarwood essential oil
5 drops tea tree essential oil

1. In a small glass bowl, add the cocoa butter and heat it in the microwave to soften.

2. Stir in the coconut oil.

3. Pierce the vitamin E capsules and squeeze the oil into the mixture.

4. Add the essential oils and mix well.

5. Transfer to an 8-ounce jar after the mixture has cooled.

APPLICATION: Rub approximately 1 teaspoon of the oil onto the affected skin.

STORAGE: Store the tightly sealed jar in a cool, dark place for up to 12 months.

CLOVE ANTI-ITCH CREAM

SCENT: SPICY/WOODY   COST: $

MAKES: APPROXIMATELY 5 OUNCES

Best known for its properties as an analgesic treatment for tooth and gum problems, clove essential oil is used in dental offices for tooth pain. It works because it contains eugenol, a substance that numbs pain at the nerve endings. Juniper is anti-inflammatory, making it an excellent itch soother.

DID YOU KNOW?

The use of the word "rash" to describe an impulsive action dates back to the 1300s, while the use of "rash" to denote a skin disorder was first used in 1709.

5 ounces (10 tablespoons) carrier oil
1 tablespoon beeswax
6 drops clove essential oil
6 drops juniper essential oil

1. Fill a small saucepan with a few inches of water and set it on the stove over low heat. Place a metal or glass bowl over the pan so that it fits well.

2. Add the carrier oil and the beeswax to the bowl and wait until the wax melts.

3. Remove the bowl from the heat and allow the mixture to cool slightly. Stir in the essential oils, using a metal spoon or a glass stirring rod.

4. Transfer the cream to a 6-ounce jar, and allow it to cool and harden before putting on the lid.

APPLICATION: Gently rub a small amount onto the affected area.

STORAGE: Store the tightly sealed jar in a cool, dark location for up to 12 months.

HIGH-PERFORMANCE BLEND MASSAGE OIL

SCENT: FLORAL/ORIENTAL   COST: $$

MAKES: 1 OUNCE

Most men who suffer from erectile dysfunction have poor blood circulation, so massaging the groin with an essential oil blend serves several functions. Physicians suggest that losing weight, getting more exercise, and stopping smoking will also help. In addition to topical treatment with essential oils, doctors often prescribe supplements such as ginkgo, astragalus, ginseng, and maca. The sensual blend in this massage oil is known to stimulate the libido of both men and women. It uses well-known aphrodisiac essential oils such as ylang ylang and sandalwood. To really set the mood, create a cocoon of scent by burning a sandalwood candle during the massage.

1 ounce sweet almond oil
6 drops ylang ylang essential oil
6 drops sandalwood essential oil

In a 1-ounce bottle, combine the almond oil with the essential oils and shake to blend.

APPLICATION: Shake before each use. Warm about a tablespoon of the blend in the palm of your hand before massaging the erogenous zone of your choice.

STORAGE: Store the tightly sealed bottle in a cool, dark place for up to 12 months.

SPICE-IT-UP BATH BLEND

SCENT: SPICY/WOODY/ORIENTAL   COST: $$

MAKES: ½ CUP

This warming, stimulating, synergistic blend can be used as a massage oil, applied as a warm compress to the groin, or poured into a warm, relaxing bath a handful at a time. Combine the essential oils without the carrier oils and add a few drops in a diffuser to set the mood. For a less expensive variation, cedarwood essential oil can be substituted for sandalwood.

½ cup carrier oil

10 drops sandalwood essential oil

10 drops ylang ylang essential oil

5 drops ginger essential oil

5 drops nutmeg essential oil

5 drops black pepper essential oil

5 drops peppermint essential oil

5 drops vetiver essential oil

In a 4-ounce bottle, combine the carrier oil with the essential oils and shake well to combine.

APPLICATION: Shake well before each use. To use as a bath oil, sprinkle 1 teaspoon into the bath as it fills.

STORAGE: Store the tightly sealed bottle in a cool, dark place for up to 12 months.

A CLOSER LOOK

In a study of 25 male medical students, Dr. Alan Hirsch of the Smell and Taste Treatment and Research Foundation in Chicago discovered that the smell of cinnamon buns increased the flow of blood to the penis.

FRANKINCENSE FLU RUB

SCENT: WOODY   COST: $$

MAKES: 1 CUP

At first glance, frankincense may seem an odd ingredient for a decongestant rub for influenza, but it has been inhaled as incense for centuries. Vitamin E is added to the blend as a natural preservative, since this recipe makes a larger quantity than many DIY projects.

SIMPLE SWAP

Substitute pine or fir needle essential oil for the cypress; both have the same decongestant properties. Pine is less expensive than cypress; fir needle is in the same price range.

¼ cup beeswax
½ cup extra-virgin coconut oil
¼ cup olive oil
3 vitamin E tablets
35 drops (½ teaspoon) frankincense essential oil
35 drops (½ teaspoon) cinnamon essential oil
35 drops (½ teaspoon) cypress essential oil

1. Fill a small saucepan with a few inches of water and set it on the stove over low heat. Place a metal or glass bowl over the pan so that it fits well.

2. Add the beeswax to the bowl and wait until it melts. Then stir in the coconut oil until it melts.

3. Remove the bowl from the heat and stir in the olive oil.

4. Pierce the vitamin E tablets and squeeze out the oil into the mixture.

5. Add the essential oils and stir with a metal spoon or glass stirring rod to combine.

6. Transfer the mixture to an 8-ounce, wide-mouth jar, and allow it to cool and harden before putting on the lid.

APPLICATION: Use 1 teaspoon to 1 tablespoon of the rub on your chest once or twice a day for congestion and cough associated with influenza.

STORAGE: Store the tightly sealed jar in a cool, dark location for 12 to 24 months.

SANITIZING HAND GEL

SCENT: MEDICINAL   COST: $

MAKES: 1 OUNCE

One of the best ways to prevent the spread of the flu virus is to wash your hands frequently. When water isn't available, sanitizing gel will do in a pinch. This gel hand sanitizer is not as harsh as the alcohol-based preparations commercially available but is effective in preventing the spread of flu bugs because it contains antibacterial essential oils, tea tree and lemon.

1 ounce aloe vera gel
6 drops tea tree essential oil
6 drops lemon essential oil

In a 1-ounce bottle, combine the aloe vera gel and the essential oils and mix with a metal stir rod.

APPLICATION: Use as needed, rubbing into the hands, especially if soap and water are not readily available.

STORAGE: Store the tightly sealed container in a cool, dry location for up to 12 months.

SIMPLE SWAP

For added anti-germ action, reduce the amount of tea tree and lemon essential oils and add up to 6 drops of eucalyptus, rosemary, or peppermint oil (or any combination of the three) to the mixture, making sure that there are no more than a total of 12 drops of essential oil per ounce of gel.

LAVENDER–EUCALYPTUS DIFFUSER BLEND

SCENT: FLORAL/MEDICINAL   COST: $

MAKES: 1 APPLICATION

This is an unusual combination of aromas, but it somehow works. The stress-relieving properties of lavender work synergistically with the mentholated scent of the eucalyptus to melt away tension. When diluted with two tablespoons of a carrier oil, this combination also works as a topical treatment when rubbed onto the temples.

A CLOSER LOOK

You may be able to stave off a full-blown migraine if you soak your hands and/or feet in a basin of hot water at the first sign that a headache's coming. Add a few drops of lavender or peppermint essential oil to the water for additional relief. Other essential oils useful for treating headaches are ginger, lemongrass, patchouli, and clove.

4 drops lavender essential oil
3 drops eucalyptus essential oil

Follow the directions for use of essential oils that come with your diffuser.

APPLICATION: Use as directed in your diffuser, or combine with an ounce of carrier oil and put in a roller bottle for topical use.

STORAGE: If using topically, store in the tightly sealed roller bottle in a cool, dark place for up to 12 months.

PEPPERMINT-LEMON HEADACHE OIL

SCENT: MINT/CITRUS   COST: $

MAKES: 1 OUNCE

This is a variation of the familiar peppermint/orange pairing that is known to reduce stress. Stress worsens tension headaches, so reducing it goes a long way toward relieving headache pain. Unless your headache has really settled in, it may be gone in as quickly as 30 minutes if you use this blend.

1 ounce carrier oil
6 drops lemon essential oil
5 drops peppermint essential oil

In a 1-ounce bottle with a roller top, combine the carrier oil with the essential oils, and shake to blend.

APPLICATION: Shake before each use. Roll onto the forehead and the back of the neck as needed.

STORAGE: Store the bottle in a cool, dark location for up to 12 months.

DID YOU KNOW?

You instinctively rub your temples when you have a headache, which is also where you should rub this oil. But that's not the only place to put the power of peppermint to work. Rub this blend on your forehead, on the back of the neck at the hairline, behind the ears, on the pulse points of the wrist, and even on the soles of your feet.

FOUR-OIL HEMORRHOID BLEND

SCENT: FLORAL/CITRUS   COST: $

MAKES: 4 TREATMENTS

Commonly known as "piles," this painful condition is the result of swollen veins in the anal canal. Hemorrhoids can be both external and internal, and both can occur at the same time. Blood in the stool is one symptom of hemorrhoids, as is rectal pain. This gentle gel-based ointment is soothing, anti-inflammatory, and healing.

A CLOSER LOOK

Hemorrhoids are basically varicose veins of the anus. They are caused when extra pressure is put on the hemorrhoidal veins, usually due to straining while passing a bowel movement. Both constipation and chronic diarrhea can aggravate hemorrhoids, as can pregnancy, obesity, or a low-fiber diet.

4 ounces witch hazel
8 drops geranium essential oil
8 drops bergamot essential oil
8 drops lavender essential oil
8 drops tea tree essential oil

In a 4-ounce spray bottle, combine the witch hazel with the essential oils.

APPLICATION: Shake the bottle well before using. Before spraying the mixture to the affected area, make sure it's clean and dry. Then spray liberally.

STORAGE: Store the capped spray bottle in a cool, dark location for up to 12 months.

SOOTHING HEMORRHOID TREATMENT

SCENT: ORIENTAL   COST: $$

MAKES: 1 OUNCE

To combat the pain and itch of hemorrhoids, sitz baths and analgesic ointments are helpful. But if the condition has progressed, and the analgesic ointments don't dull the pain, you will need something a little stronger. This preparation is filled with oils whose therapeutic qualities have been known for centuries. If the condition worsens or does not seem to be getting better, consult a health care professional. Hemorrhoids are painful but rarely dangerous.

1 ounce carrier oil
10 drops lavender essential oil
10 drops frankincense essential oil
10 drops cypress essential oil
5 drops geranium essential oil
5 drops sandalwood essential oil

In a 2-ounce bottle, combine the essential oils with the carrier oil and shake to mix.

APPLICATION: Shake before using. Apply 5 to 6 drops to the affected area as needed, no more than 3 times per day.

STORAGE: Store the tightly sealed bottle in a cool, dry location for up to 12 months.

DID YOU KNOW?

Napoleon Bonaparte suffered from hemorrhoids and, according to historical records, the condition was so painful he could barely sit on his horse during the Battle of Waterloo.

ANTISEPTIC SPRAY

SCENT: CITRUS/MEDICINAL   COST: $

MAKES: 4 OUNCES

"Infection" is another one of those umbrella phrases that applies to conditions caused by all sorts of organisms. An infection can be bacterial, viral, fungal, or parasitic. Some of these conditions are benign, others are life threatening. Not every infection responds to the same treatment, but everyone should have an all-purpose antiseptic spray in their home medicine cabinet. Many essential oils have antibacterial and antiseptic properties and can be substituted for those in this recipe.

TIP

In a pinch, diluting a little rosemary or oregano essential oil with some olive oil and smoothing it right on a cut or rash will work.

4 ounces carrier oil

3 drops orange essential oil

3 drops lavender essential oil

3 drops eucalyptus essential oil

3 drops tea tree essential oil

In a 4-ounce spray bottle, combine the carrier oil with the essential oils and shake well to combine.

APPLICATION: Shake before each use. Spray on cuts, scrapes, and rashes as needed.

STORAGE: Store the tightly sealed bottle in a cool, dry location for up to 12 months.

ABSCESS-RELIEVING COMPRESS

SCENT: MEDICINAL/FLORAL   COST: $

MAKES: 1 TREATMENT

Abscesses are pockets of infection that can be quite painful. This soothing hot compress serves several functions. First, the tea tree and lavender essential oils have antibiotic properties that can help with the infection in the abscess. Additionally, the heat of the compress can help the abscess drain on its own. If you have an abscess that is particularly painful or has a red streak going from it, see your doctor right away.

⅓ cup hot water
4 drops tea tree essential oil
4 drops lavender essential oil

In a small metal or glass bowl, combine the water and essential oils, mixing well.

APPLICATION: Soak a washcloth in the hot-water mixture. Place the hot compress on the affected area for 15 minutes every 2 to 3 hours.

STORAGE: This is a single-use treatment and should be discarded after each application.

LAVENDER–TEA TREE LICE TREATMENT

SCENT: FLORAL/MEDICINAL/SPICY   COST: $

MAKES: 1 TREATMENT

If you have school-aged children you live with the persistent threat that one of them may come home with head lice. This hair treatment is only one aspect of removing lice. You also need to remove all of the nits, and wash all bedding, linens, and clothing in hot water. Tea tree and lavender essential oils have antibacterial properties that will help remove the lice and nits. The other essential oils will also help kill the pests and, if used properly, prevent recurrence.

NOTE

Tea tree oil and lavender must always be diluted before being applied topically. Tea tree oil is a powerful insecticide.

FOR THE LICE LOTION

1 ounce aloe vera gel

15 drops lavender essential oil

15 drops tea tree essential oil

12 drops thyme essential oil

4 drops clove essential oil

1 drop cinnamon leaf essential oil

FOR THE NIT REMOVAL BLEND

1 gallon of water

10 drops tea tree essential oil

TO MAKE THE LICE LOTION

In a small bowl or 4-ounce bottle, combine the aloe vera gel with the essential oils, and shake to mix well.

TO MAKE THE NIT REMOVAL BLEND

In an extra-large glass or metal mixing bowl or a 2-gallon bucket, mix together the ingredients.

APPLICATION

1. Massage the Lice Lotion onto the scalp, making sure it coats all of the hair. Cover the head with a shower cap and leave the cap on for 8 hours (overnight).
2. Shampoo the hair and rinse.
3. Use a lice comb or fine-tooth comb to remove the nits. Dip the comb frequently into the Nit Removal Blend to remove the nits from the comb's teeth. Shampoo the hair again.
4. Dry the hair and comb through to look for nits again.
5. Repeat the entire process every 2 days for 2 to 3 weeks.

STORAGE: This is a single-use treatment.

ANTIFUNGAL LOTION FOR RINGWORM

SCENT: CITRUS/FLORAL/HERBAL   COST: $

MAKES: 1 OUNCE

Ringworm is itchy and highly contagious. It occurs as a result of a fungal infection. All of the essential oils in this blend exhibit antifungal properties, which is why this mixture is so effective at combating ringworm. The lavender essential oil is also soothing and can calm the itch associated with ringworm rash.

SIMPLE SWAP

Some rarer essential oils are especially effective at fighting ringworm if you're dealing with a very serious outbreak. Consider using myrrh, tea tree, palmarosa, or manuka essential oils, concentrating them at a mix of 1 drop of essential oil to 1 teaspoon of carrier oil.

1 ounce carrier oil

2 drops lemon essential oil

2 drops rosemary essential oil

2 drops basil essential oil

2 drops lavender essential oil

2 drops tea tree essential oil

In a 1-ounce bottle, combine the carrier oil with the essential oils and shake to blend.

APPLICATION: Wash the rash with soap and water. Dry thoroughly. Shake the bottle before each use and dab a small amount of the lotion around the edges of the lesions rather than directly on the ringworm.

STORAGE: Store the tightly sealed bottle in a cool, dark location for up to 12 months.

NO SWEAT MIST

SCENT: MINTY/FLORAL   COST: $

MAKES: 1 OUNCE

Hot flashes occur as a result of hormonal imbalances arising during perimenopause and menopause. This blend helps to balance the hormones and provide cooling during hot flashes. The peppermint is especially good at helping cool the skin's surface when hot flashes occur, and the cool water helps as well. Keep the mixture in the refrigerator for even more cooling action.

DID YOU KNOW?

The world's oldest surviving medical text, the *Kahun Gynaecological Papyrus* (c. 1800 BCE), is a treatise on women's health, particularly female reproductive health. A number of remedies are prescribed for various conditions of the womb, including massage of the stomach with "one *hin* (about 1.6 gallons) of fresh oil" and inhalation of incense.

4 ounces distilled water

1 teaspoon vodka

20 drops clary sage essential oil

20 drops geranium essential oil

20 drops peppermint essential oil

In a 4-ounce spray bottle, combine the water and vodka with the essential oils, and shake well to mix.

APPLICATION: Shake before each use. Spritz the blend all over the face and body to cool down a hot flash.

STORAGE: Store the spray bottle in the refrigerator for up to 12 months.

HORMONE HELP BATH

SCENT: WOODY/CITRUS   COST: $$

MAKES: ½ CUP

Many of the changes in menopause occur as hormones move out of balance. A soothing bath is the perfect way to relax and escape from some of the hormonally induced anxieties that come with menopause. Add the blend to your bath every other day to let the properties of the essential oils help balance your menopausal hormones.

½ cup carrier oil
15 drops clary sage essential oil
12 drops bergamot essential oil
12 drops geranium essential oil

In a 4-ounce bottle, combine the carrier oil with the essential oils and shake well to blend.

APPLICATION: Add 2 tablespoons of the mixture to running bath water. Soak for 15 minutes.

STORAGE: Store the tightly sealed bottle in a cool, dark place for up to 12 months.

SIMPLE SWAP

You can also use the essential oils in a spray: Omit the carrier oil and replace it with ½ cup of water and 1 teaspoon vodka, shaking well to mix. Store in a spray bottle in the refrigerator and spritz on your face and body as needed.

SPEARMINT ANTI-NAUSEA DROPS

SCENT: MINTY/CITRUS   COST: $

MAKES: 1 TEASPOON

Rub this refreshing topical blend on pulse points to relieve morning sickness. However, you need to give your body a break from this blend occasionally, so don't use for more than five days in a row before taking at least two days off. The spearmint and lemon essential oils are safe during pregnancy and have calming digestive effects.

DID YOU KNOW?

When Kate Middleton, the Duchess of Cambridge, was pregnant with her first child, she had terrible morning sickness. In an attempt to find relief, she turned to aromatherapy candles made from the essential oil of the buchu, a plant native to South Africa with a scent similar to blackcurrant. While the scent worked for her, you should consult with a licensed aromatherapist, as some of the chemical constituents of the oil are identical to those in pennyroyal, which is extremely toxic.

1 teaspoon carrier oil
1 drop spearmint essential oil
1 drop lemon essential oil

1. Measure 1 teaspoon of carrier oil onto a shallow saucer.

2. Add the drops of essential oil.

3. Stir with a clean finger.

APPLICATION: Dab the oil onto the skin at the wrists and other pulse points.

STORAGE: This is a single-use treatment and does not require storage.

GINGER LOTION

SCENT: SPICY/CITRUS   COST: $

MAKES: 1 OUNCE

Gingerroot has long been used in many forms to ease nausea. It can be drunk as a tea or soft drink, eaten in its pickled or candied forms, or added to food and drink in its powdered or grated form. This spicy, warming oil blend is perfect for massaging onto the skin on wrists, at the back of the knees, and at other pulse points. This lotion is also effective for the nausea associated with motion sickness.

1 ounce carrier oil
4 drops ginger essential oil
2 drops orange essential oil

In a 1-ounce bottle, combine the carrier oil with the essential oils and shake to blend.

APPLICATION: Shake before using. Apply to pulse points no more than twice per day.

STORAGE: Store the tightly sealed bottle in a cool, dry location in an airtight container for up to 12 months.

REJUVENATING JUNIPER BATH SOAK

SCENT: WOODY/CITRUS   COST: $

MAKES: ¾ CUP

This reviving soak combines the anti-inflammatory properties of the lemon with the detoxifying elements from the juniper berry. The natural minerals in the sea salt also provide relaxation, making this bath soak both soothing and stimulating.

DID YOU KNOW?

Juniper essential oil is sometimes adulterated with oil of turpentine, a volatile oil distilled from pine resin or other evergreen trees.

½ cup sea salt
¼ cup jojoba oil
4 drops lemon essential oil
3 drops juniper essential oil

1. In a small glass bowl, mix together the salt and the jojoba oil.

2. Add the essential oils and mix well.

3. Transfer the mixture to a 6-ounce bottle or jar.

APPLICATION: Use 2 tablespoons per bath, swirling it into the warm bath water. Soak for 15 to 20 minutes.

STORAGE: Store the tightly sealed container in a cool, dark place for up to 12 months.

PALMAROSA PMS MASSAGE OIL

SCENT: FLORAL/CITRUS COST: $$

MAKES: 1 OUNCE

Premenstrual syndrome is the name given to the hormonal changes in the week to ten days before a woman's menstrual cycle begins. Symptoms can vary widely, from physical manifestations like acne and bloating, to anxiety, mood swings, inability to concentrate, and depression. The rosehip oil in this formula is particularly soothing to stressed skin and works well with the rosy notes of the palmarosa and geranium. A woman's sense of smell is often heightened just before her period, and this fragrance is soothing.

SIMPLE SWAP

If you don't have bergamot essential oil, you can replace it with grapefruit, orange, or mandarin essential oils.

1 ounce rosehip oil

3 drops palmarosa essential oil

3 drops geranium essential oil

3 drops bergamot essential oil

In a 1-ounce bottle, combine the rosehip oil with the essential oils and shake to blend.

APPLICATION: Shake well before each use. Use 1 tablespoon as a massage oil during times of PMS.

STORAGE: Store the tightly sealed bottle in a cool, dry place for up to 12 months.

PMS BLEND VOTIVE CANDLE

SCENT: FLORAL COST: $

MAKES: 6 VOTIVE CANDLES

Burn these mood-elevating candles to help soothe the irritability that often arrives before your period. You can safely add up to 1 ounce of essential oil and up to 1 pound of beeswax, but no more. An over-fragranced candle will smoke when burning.

---

5 (3-ounce) wax-coated, flat-bottomed paper cups

6 candle wicks

14 ounces beeswax

10 drops liquid candle dye (optional)

2 teaspoons lavender essential oil

2 teaspoons geranium essential oil

1. Put the wax paper cups on a cookie sheet to keep melted wax from getting on your counter.

2. Hang the wicks, weighted side down, in the middle of each cup. To keep the wicks vertical, wrap the loose end around a pencil or chopstick balanced across the center of the mouth of the cup.

3. Fill a small saucepan with a few inches of water and set it on the stove over low heat. Place a metal or glass bowl over the pan so that it fits well.

4. Add the beeswax to the bowl and wait until it melts. Use a candy thermometer to monitor the heat of the melting wax. When the wax reaches 170°F, remove the bowl from the heat and stir in the candle dye, blending the color, if using.

5. Stir in the essential oils using a metal spoon or glass stirring rod.

6. Pour the melted wax into the paper cups, making sure to leave a little space at the top of the cups. Note: Do not discard the remaining wax or over-fill your "molds."

7. Allow the candles to harden. The wax will shrink as it cools and may leave a dip in the center of the candle.

8. When the candles have cooled, reheat the leftover wax and pour another layer over the top of the hardened layer.

9. Let the candles stand until solid. This will take about 5 hours.

10. Trim the wick to between ¼ and ½ inch.

11. Tear away the paper cup mold.

APPLICATION: Burn a candle when you are in the same room with it to relieve PMS.

STORAGE: Store the candles in a cool, dry location for up to 24 months.

DIFFUSER BLENDS THAT HELP SAD

SCENT: DEPENDS ON THE BLEND   COST: $–$$

MAKES: 1 TREATMENT

The scent-mood connection comes into play with inhalation therapy for the stresses and sadness that are triggered by changes in season. These blends have proven to be particularly effective. Use as directed for your diffuser.

DID YOU KNOW?

Most people associate the mood disorder Seasonal Affective Disorder (SAD) with the rainy, gray, and cold days of fall and winter. In fact, there's a lesser-known kind of SAD, known as "summer depression," that is believed to be triggered by heat and humidity rather than lack of light.

CITRUS-JUNIPER BLEND

2 drops grapefruit essential oil

2 drops juniper essential oil

2 drops bergamot essential oil or 1 drop orange essential oil

CALMING CHAMOMILE BLEND

2 drops lavender essential oil

2 drops lemon essential oil

2 drops chamomile essential oil

ROSY FUTURE BLEND

3 drops palmarosa essential oil

2 drops bergamot essential oil or orange essential oil

Combine the oils in a small container and use in a diffuser or oil burner.

APPLICATION: Use the blend in a diffuser, following the directions for your specific diffuser.

STORAGE: Each is a single-use application so no storage is necessary.

MOOD ELEVATING SPRITZ

SCENT: CITRUS   COST: $

MAKES: 2 OUNCES

Scent has been proven to elevate mood. Bright, sunny, citrusy scents are particularly mood elevating. While this spritz uses a single scent to keep from getting muddled, you can substitute essential oils in the citrus family in place of the bergamot. Then, when you're feeling down, spritz the air around you with a little bit of this liquid sunshine.

SIMPLE SWAP

The bergamot essential oil can be substituted with an equal amount of grapefruit, sweet orange, mandarin, or lemon essential oils.

2 ounces water

1 teaspoon vodka

24 drops bergamot essential oil

In a 3-ounce spray bottle, combine the water and vodka with the essential oil and shake well.

APPLICATION: Shake well before each use. Spritz into the air twice per day to relieve mild depression associated with SAD.

STORAGE: Store, tightly sealed, in the spray bottle in a cool, dry location for up to 12 months.

EUCALYPTUS–SANDALWOOD SINUS RELIEF

SCENT: SPICY/ORIENTAL   COST: $$

MAKES: 1 OUNCE

Sinus pain is the result of a build-up of pressure in the sinuses of a skull. This usually occurs when the sinus becomes inflamed as the result of an allergic reaction, congestion, or infection. Hot compresses are known to relieve the pain, and staying hydrated helps also. This is a thermogenic blend that will heat the skin slightly as the aromatic essential oils work their magic.

1 ounce sweet almond oil
9 drops sandalwood essential oil
3 drops eucalyptus essential oil

In a small bottle with a roller top, combine the sweet almond oil and the essential oils, and shake to blend.

APPLICATION: Shake well before each use. Apply to the bridge of the nose and right beside the nostrils, gently massaging each point to ease the pressure.

STORAGE: Store in an airtight roller bottle in a cool, dark location for up to 12 months.

SIMPLE SWAP

If sandalwood essential oil is too expensive, replace it with cedarwood essential oil.

SINUS-SOOTHING DIFFUSER BLEND

SCENT: WOODY/FLORAL/MEDICINAL   COST: $

MAKES: 1 APPLICATION

This blend not only has medicinal properties, but the lavender also brings about relaxation while the pine and other essential oils invigorate. Use it in your diffuser. It also works well in a bowl of steam. Just drape a towel over your head to trap the steam and breathe it in for five to ten minutes.

2 drops lavender essential oil

1 drop pine essential oil

1 drop tea tree essential oil

1 drop eucalyptus essential oil

1 drop rosemary essential oil

In a small glass bowl, combine all of the essential oils.

APPLICATION: Follow the directions that come with your diffuser.

STORAGE: This is a single-dose application, so no storage is required.

SIMPLE SWAP

If you don't have most of the essential oils required for this recipe, it's easy to make using just eucalyptus and lavender essential oils instead. To make the blend with these two ingredients, use 3 drops of lavender essential oil and 3 drops of eucalyptus oil.

CHAMOMILE SUNBURN GEL

SCENT: FLORAL   COST: $

MAKES: ¼ CUP

Aloe vera gel has long been prized for its burn-healing, cooling, and soothing properties. It also moisturizes to protect sunburned skin from damage. The gel can be squeezed directly from the plant and used to soothe a burn. The chamomile adds a pleasant floral scent, and it won't irritate sensitive burned skin.

DID YOU KNOW?

American pioneers treated severe sunburn by covering the burns with poultices of cold, cooked oatmeal.

¼ cup (2 ounces) pure aloe vera gel
6 drops chamomile essential oil

In a 2-ounce jar, combine the gel and essential oil. Stir with a metal rod to mix.

APPLICATION: Smooth 1 to 2 tablespoons on burned areas.

STORAGE: Store the tightly sealed jar in a cool, dry location for up to 12 months. For even more cooling power, store the gel in the refrigerator.

COOLING SUNBURN SPRITZ

SCENT: FLORAL   COST: $

MAKES: ABOUT 2 OUNCES

Your best defense against sunburn is protection—using sunscreen, staying in the shade, or wearing sun-blocking clothing. However, sometimes you get burned in spite of your best intentions. When that happens, this cooling spray combines the soothing power of aloe vera with peppermint essential oil, which is excellent at soothing minor burns and itching. For even more cooling power, store it in the refrigerator and pull it out whenever your sunburn becomes irritated or itchy.

1½ ounces distilled water
½ ounce aloe vera gel
4 drops peppermint essential oil

In a 2-ounce spray bottle, combine all the ingredients and shake well to mix.

APPLICATION: Shake well before using. Spray on sunburned areas once or twice per day.

STORAGE: Store the tightly sealed spray bottle in a cool, dark place for up to 12 months. Store in the refrigerator for more cooling action.

MYRRH MOUTHWASH FOR TOOTHACHE

SCENT: SPICY   COST: $$

MAKES: 1 CUP

Anyone who complains about a baby crying when he or she is teething has never suffered the pain of an impacted wisdom tooth. Wisdom teeth are the last adult teeth to emerge in the mouth and they become impacted when they don't erupt as they are supposed to. This mouthwash contains clove oil, which dentists still use in their practices to dull nerve pain.

1 cup distilled water
2 drops myrrh essential oil
2 drops clove essential oil
1 drop lavender essential oil

In an 8-ounce bottle, combine all the ingredients and shake well to combine.

APPLICATION: Use as necessary to relieve pain, swishing 1 to 2 tablespoons in the mouth for 30 to 60 seconds. Do not swallow the rinse.

STORAGE: Store the tightly sealed bottle in a cool, dark place for up to 12 months.

THE TAMANU–TEA TREE BATH

SCENT: MEDICINAL   COST: $

MAKES: 1 TREATMENT

A urinary tract infection (UTI) is a common bacterial infection that is often characterized by pain or a burning sensation during urination, the constant need to urinate, and dark or cloudy urine. Symptoms may also include fever and pain in the sides. Tea tree essential oil is particularly effective for the treatment of urinary tract infections due to its antibacterial properties.

2 teaspoons tamanu oil
4 drops tea tree essential oil

In a small bowl, add the tamanu oil and then the tea tree essential oil. Mix well. Then add the mixture to a warm bath.

APPLICATION: Soak in the bath for at least 15 minutes.

STORAGE: This is a single-use treatment and should not be stored.

DID YOU KNOW?

Folk wisdom has long held that drinking cranberry juice can help heal UTI, but a review by the Cochrane Collaboration, an independent, non-profit, nongovernmental organization dedicated to organizing evidence-based medical research, found that the juice had little, if any, benefit and could in fact cause gastrointestinal upset in 30 percent of patients. Other research suggests that cranberries and blueberries contain substances that do, indeed, prevent bacteria from adhering to the urinary tract, possibly preventing UTI.

THE MEDICINAL COMPRESS

SCENT: CITRUS/FLORAL   COST: $$

MAKES: 1 COMPRESS

If you have a UTI that does not respond within a few days to home treatment, such as drinking lots of water and eating raw garlic, see a doctor. UTIs can be serious and may require medical intervention. This warm compress will help soothe the burning and discomfort associated with urinary tract infections.

SIMPLE SWAP

If you don't have sandalwood or it is too expensive, replace it with cedarwood.

3 drops bergamot essential oil
2 drops lavender essential oil
2 drops chamomile essential oil
1 drop sandalwood essential oil

1. Use a washcloth or small towel for your compress. Pull up the stopper in the sink and put the compress at the bottom of the sink, then fill it with hot water.

2. Add the essential oils and swish around to blend. Drain the sink.

3. Allow the compress to get fully soaked and then remove from the sink and wring out.

APPLICATION: Apply the hot compress to the lower abdomen or above the kidneys once or twice a day to relieve pain.

STORAGE: This is a single-use treatment and should not be stored. Use right away. Repeat the directions to make a new compress for each use.

TWISTED SISTER VARICOSE VEIN BODY BUTTER

SCENT: CITRUS/HERBAL   COST: $

MAKES: APPROXIMATELY 1 CUP

This body butter combines circulation-boosting grapefruit essential oil with the anti-inflammatory power of lavender essential oil for a one-two punch to flatten veins. The recipe is very customizable. Other essential oils that stimulate circulation include lemon, lime, and rosemary. Swap chamomile, marjoram, or peppermint for the lavender essential oil.

SIMPLE SWAP

For a different fragrance with the same properties, swap the lavender for chamomile essential oil and the grapefruit for bergamot essential oil.

½ cup shea butter
½ cup carrier oil
3 vitamin E capsules
15 drops grapefruit essential oil
15 drops lavender essential oil

1. In a medium glass bowl, melt the shea butter in the microwave, using 10-second bursts.

2. Stir in the carrier oil.

3. Pierce the vitamin E capsules and squeeze the oil into the shea butter mix.

4. Add the essential oils and stir well.

5. Chill the mixture for 90 minutes.

6. Remove from the refrigerator and, using a hand mixer, whip the body butter until it is smooth and creamy.

7. Transfer to an 8-ounce glass jar.

APPLICATION: Using gentle strokes, apply body butter on legs and arms, always stroking toward the heart.

STORAGE: Store the tightly sealed jar in a cool, dry place for up to 12 months.

VARICOSE VEIN MASSAGE OIL BLENDS

SCENT: VARIES   COST: $–$$

MAKES: 4 OUNCES

To achieve relief from varicose veins, gently massage one of these blends around the veins, but not directly on them. Use light strokes moving in the direction of the heart. Each of these blends begins with 4 ounces of carrier oil, to which 24 drops of essential oil have been added. These blends are believed to work synergistically.

GERANIUM–CYPRESS BLEND

4 ounces carrier oil

12 drops geranium essential oil

12 drops cypress essential oil

ROSEMARY–CHAMOMILE BLEND

4 ounces carrier oil

9 drops chamomile essential oil

15 drops rosemary essential oil

TEA TREE–THYME BLEND

4 ounces carrier oil

12 drops tea tree essential oil

12 drops thyme essential oil

In a small bottle, combine all the ingredients for your specific blend, and shake well.

APPLICATION: Massage around varicose veins once or twice per day.

STORAGE: Store, tightly sealed, in a cool, dry place for up to 12 months.

TEA TREE INTERNAL SALVE

SCENT: MEDICINAL   COST: $

MAKES: 1 TREATMENT

This method is a refinement of the suppository treatment, in which medicine is mixed with a solid for insertion into the vagina or rectum. In this case, a tampon serves as the suppository while tea tree oil's antifungal action fights the yeast overgrowth.

1 tampon

1 tablespoon extra-virgin coconut oil

2 drops tea tree essential oil

In a small bowl, mix the coconut oil with the tea tree essential oil.

APPLICATION: With clean fingers, apply the salve to a tampon and insert directly into the vagina. Repeat treatment every 3 or 4 days, or as infection persists.

STORAGE: This is a single-use treatment and should not be stored.

YOGURT AND TEA TREE REMEDY

SCENT: MEDICINAL   COST: $

MAKES: 1 TREATMENT

The delivery system of this essential oil treatment is messy but highly effective. Yogurt will work well on its own by replenishing yeast-consuming bacteria, but the medicinal properties of tea tree essential oil work synergistically with the probiotic power of the dairy product. Eating yogurt with acidophilus may help keep the infection from recurring, but don't eat the yogurt that has tea tree oil in it. That is for vaginal insertion only.

DID YOU KNOW?

Frequent yeast infections can be a warning sign of diabetes. If you have frequent yeast infections and a family history of diabetes, consider having your blood sugar checked next time you visit your doctor.

2 tablespoons plain, unsweetened yogurt
6 drops tea tree essential oil

In a small bowl, add the yogurt and then the essential oil, and mix well.

APPLICATION: Apply the treated yogurt directly to the inside of the vagina. (A squeeze bottle might help.) Put on a pair of high-waisted cotton panties or an adult diaper to help absorb any of the remedy that may not stay in the vagina. Leave the mixture in as long as you are able before showering the remains away.

STORAGE: This is a single-use treatment and should not be stored. Use this remedy as soon as you make it.

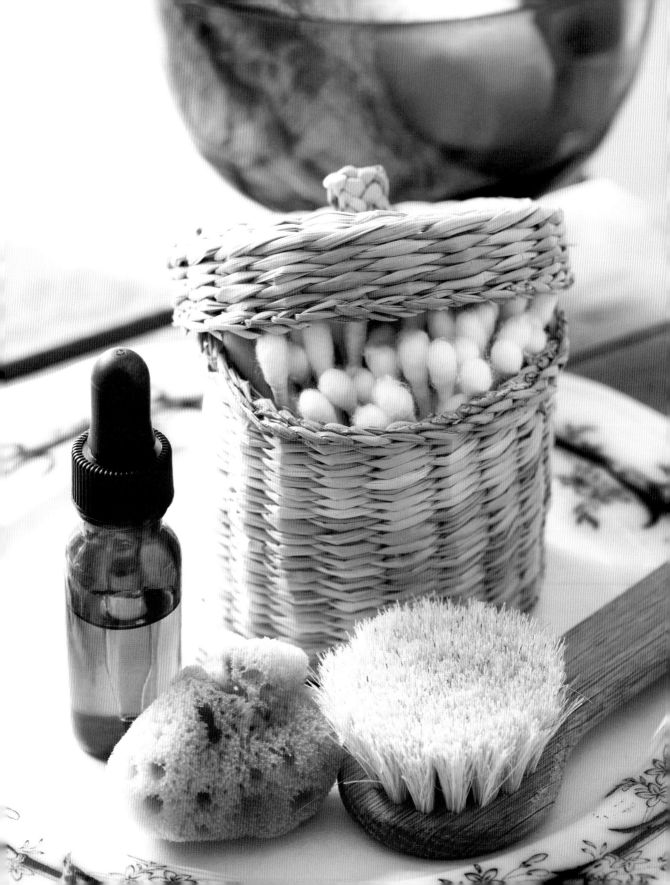

6

REMEDIES FOR COSMETIC CARE

Acne 162 Aging Skin and Skin Rejuvenation 164 Chapped Lips 165

Dry Skin 168 Exfoliation 171 Face Care 174 Hair Care 177 Hand and Foot Care 182

Nail Care 186 Rosacea 188 Stretch Marks 190

Beauty may only be skin deep, but when your cosmetics are enriched with essential oils, the benefits penetrate the skin, bringing you benefits at a deeper level. Making your own beauty products is not only fun—like playing with the best chemistry set ever—but allows you to detox your beauty routine and save money. You can also make thoughtful, personalized gifts. (DIY aromatherapy cosmetic crafting can even make you money if you have an entrepreneurial spirit.) Build on the basics and make these recipes your own.

ANTI-ACNE "SPOT NOT" MASK

SCENT: MEDICINAL   COST: $

MAKES: 1 TREATMENT

Acne breakouts can be annoying at best and disfiguring at worst. Commercial acne treatments are harsh and drying to the skin, and for people with sensitive skin they may be especially problematic. This simple facial treatment contains rosemary essential oil, which stimulates and regenerates cell growth, and thyme essential oil, which fights bacteria and infection that contributes to acne break-outs. The lactic acid in the yogurt serves as a mini peel, peeling away dead skin that may contribute to blocked pores.

SIMPLE SWAP
You can use other antibacterial oils in place of the rosemary and thyme, such as tea tree or lavender oils.

3 tablespoons (1½ ounces) full-fat unflavored yogurt
2 tablespoons organic, raw liquid honey
2 drops rosemary essential oil
2 drops thyme essential oil

In a small bowl, mix together all the ingredients.

APPLICATION:

1. Using a fan brush, apply the mixture in a thin layer to the face and allow it to dry.
2. Add a second layer to the first and allow it to dry. Continue applying layers and allowing them to dry until you have used all the honey-yogurt mixture.
3. Leave the mask on for 15 minutes. Then rinse it away with warm water and remove any stubborn spots with a washcloth.
4. Pat your face dry with a clean towel.

STORAGE: This is a single-use treatment and should not be stored.

NOURISHING NIGHTTIME LOTION

SCENT: EARTHY/CITRUS   COST: $$

MAKES: 2 OUNCES

It is a common misconception that acne-prone skin doesn't need any more lubrication. Moisturizing can help open pores, which helps prevent blemishes from forming in the first place. Avoid using alcohol-based moisturizers as they can cause inflammation. The combination of essential oils in this lotion has a clean, unisex scent, and the hazelnut oil absorbs into the skin without leaving behind excess oil.

2 ounces hazelnut oil

4 drops borage seed oil

2 drops carrot seed oil (optional)

4 drops fennel essential oil

2 drops bergamot essential oil

In a 2-ounce bottle, combine all the ingredients, and shake well.

APPLICATION: Using your fingertips, gently pat the oil into your face at bedtime.

STORAGE: Store the tightly sealed bottle in the refrigerator for up to 6 months.

SIMPLE SWAP

Sweet almond oil is another light and noncomedogenic (doesn't clog pores) carrier oil that makes an excellent substitution here. To make this a wrinkle-fighting oil, try using rosehip oil in place of the borage oil.

FRANKINCENSE AND COMMON SENSE SERUM

SCENT: ORIENTAL   COST: $$

MAKES: 2 OUNCES

"Age cannot wither her," said Mark Antony of Cleopatra, who knew a thing or two about beauty. Frankincense has been used since ancient times as a skin conditioner, and this richly fragrant serum is healing and restorative. The evening primrose oil and vitamin E also add to the antiaging properties of this serum, while the carrot and geranium essential oils boost the serum's antioxidants.

2½ tablespoons sweet almond oil
½ tablespoon jojoba oil
2 drops evening primrose oil
2 drops vitamin E oil
2 drops carrot seed essential oil
10 drops frankincense essential oil
10 drops geranium essential oil
10 drops cypress essential oil

In a 2-ounce bottle, combine all the ingredients and stir to combine.

APPLICATION: Use fingertips to smooth the serum over the face and neck nightly before going to bed.

STORAGE: Store, tightly sealed, in the refrigerator for up to 6 months.

NOTE

Evening primrose oil is very delicate and breaks down easily, so this formulation won't last as long as something containing a different type of oil. However, the vitamin E helps preserve it, so it will last a little longer. Discard the mixture if it smells odd or looks discolored.

BASIC LIP BALM

SCENT: YOUR CHOICE   COST: $

MAKES: 1 OUNCE

Lips can chap and crack easily, especially during extreme weather. Having an effective lip balm can help prevent cracking and chapping and soothe sore lips that have become chapped. This lip balm recipe uses moisturizing coconut oil to protect and soothe your lips.

NOTE
If you prefer a harder texture for your lip balm, double the amount of beeswax in the recipe.

3 teaspoons grated beeswax
3 teaspoons extra-virgin coconut oil
5 drops essential oil

1. Fill a small saucepan with a few inches of water and set it on the stove over low heat. Place a metal or glass bowl over the pan so that it fits well. Add the beeswax to the bowl and wait until it melts. Then stir in the coconut oil.

2. Remove the bowl from the heat and stir in the essential oil using a metal spoon or glass stirring rod.

3. Transfer the mixture to a 1-ounce jar, tin, or chosen container, and allow the lip balm to harden.

4. The balm may settle as it hardens. Top it off with more melted balm and allow it to harden for 10 minutes before using.

APPLICATION: Smooth over your lips with a finger 2 or 3 times per day.

STORAGE: Store the container in a cool, dark location for up to 12 months. Or toss it in your purse, and it will last for about 6 months.

LEMON-LAVENDER LIP BALM

SCENT: FLORAL/CITRUS   COST: $

MAKES: 1 OUNCE

Once you see how easy and affordable it is to make your own lip balm, you'll enjoy making additional batches for friends and family. Store it in lip balm tins (even breath mint tins would work), small jars, or new or recycled lip balm tubes. This recipe uses fragrant lemon and lavender to soothe and protect lips, but you can play with your own scents.

SIMPLE SWAP

For a nourishing and spicy-scented variation, make ginger–ylang ylang lip balm by substituting ginger and ylang ylang essential oils for the lemon and lavender. Equal parts iris and geranium essential oils can also be substituted for the lavender and lemon essential oils.

3 teaspoons grated beeswax
3 teaspoons extra-virgin coconut oil
5 drops lemon essential oil
5 drops lavender essential oil

1. Fill a small saucepan with a few inches of water and set it on the stove over low heat. Place a metal or glass bowl over the pan so that it fits well.

2. Add the beeswax to the bowl and wait until it melts. Then stir in the coconut oil.

3. Remove the bowl from the heat and stir in the essential oils using a metal spoon or glass stirring rod.

4. Pour the mixture into lip balm tubes or tins quickly, before it hardens. The balm may settle as it hardens. If it does, add more and allow it to harden for 10 minutes before using.

APPLICATION: Smooth a dab of the lip balm over your lips as needed throughout the day.

STORAGE: Store the unused, tightly sealed containers of the lip balm for up to 12 months in a cool, dark location. Opened containers will last for up to 6 months in your purse.

GERANIUM LIP SCRUB

SCENT: FLORAL   COST: $

MAKES: APPROXIMATELY 3 OUNCES

Pretty, healthy lips require a little exfoliation every now and then to remove dry skin and reveal smooth new skin. This easy sugar scrub sweetly removes dry skin from the lips and moisturizes with coconut oil and geranium essential oil.

GIFT IT

Pair this lip scrub with a lip balm and you have a great DIY gift for a birthday or another occasion. Slip them into a goodie bag or stuff them in a stocking. Keep one for yourself and stash it at the office for use when winter weather has done its worst.

2 tablespoons extra-virgin coconut oil
2 tablespoons honey
2 tablespoons granulated sugar
6 drops geranium essential oil

1. In a small bowl, combine the coconut oil and honey. Whip until smooth.

2. Add the granulated sugar and essential oil and stir to combine.

3. Transfer the mixture to a 3-ounce bottle or jar.

APPLICATION: To use, apply to the lips with a fingertip and rub in for a minute. Let the scrub sit for another 5 minutes before gently wiping the lips with a warm washcloth.

STORAGE: Store the tightly sealed container in a cool, dark location for up to 12 months.

SANDALWOOD SERUM

SCENT: WOODY/CITRUS   COST: $$

MAKES: 1 OUNCE

Next to exfoliation, the other secret to treating dry skin is keeping it hydrated and moisturized. The exotic scent of this luxurious wrinkle cream will connect you to an ageless past. Use this serum in addition to your regular moisturizers to boost the effectiveness of both in areas that need a little extra help.

SIMPLE SWAP

Either bergamot or the less expensive orange essential oil work for this mix, as sandalwood blends well with a number of citrus oils. Note that the citrus oils are phototoxic, so stay out of the sun after applying this serum.

1 tablespoon rosehip oil
1 tablespoon sweet almond oil
10 drops sandalwood essential oil
2 drops lemon essential oil

In a 1-ounce bottle, combine the oils with the essential oils and shake to blend.

APPLICATION: Shake before using. Smooth 1 to 2 drops on your face at bedtime before moisturizing. Allow the serum to settle into the skin for a minute or so before applying moisturizer.

STORAGE: Rosehip oil spoils quickly, so make very small batches of this serum and keep it tightly sealed in the refrigerator for 3 to 6 months. If it develops an off smell, discard it.

BASIC BODY BUTTER

SCENT: YOUR CHOICE   COST: $

MAKES: YOUR CHOICE

"Body butter" is a marketing term that basically means a heavy moisturizer meant to be used on the body rather than the face, where it might clog pores and cause acne. Body butters are usually built around a base of a solid carrier such as shea butter, coconut oil, or mango butter, which is a product cold-pressed from mango seeds that has much the same properties as cocoa butter.

TIP

Shea butter is solid, but soft at room temperature. Refined shea butter is sold in health food groceries like Whole Foods, but for the pure, unrefined product, you can order it from Mountain Rose Herbs or Butters and Bars (see Resources).

½ cup shea butter
2 tablespoons sweet almond oil
20 drops essential oil

1. In a medium bowl, mix the shea butter and the almond oil with a fork.

2. Add the essential oil of your choosing and mix well.

3. To make the texture creamier, whip the mixture with a hand mixer for 6 to 10 minutes to "fluff" it up.

4. Transfer to a 5-ounce jar.

APPLICATION: Smooth liberally on dry skin once or twice per day.

STORAGE: Store the tightly sealed jar in a cool, dark place for up to 12 months.

CITRUS-FLOWER BODY BUTTER

SCENT: CITRUS/FLORAL   COST: $$

MAKES: 1 CUP

The sweet floral notes of the ylang ylang essential oil pair well with the soft orange scent of neroli essential oil to create a light, fragrant, and nourishing body butter. Smooth it on all over the body after a bath when the skin more readily absorbs moisture from lotions and butters.

SIMPLE SWAP

Neroli essential oil can be pricey, so feel free to substitute it with sweet orange, mandarin, or any other low-cost citrus oil.

½ cup sweet almond oil
½ cup extra-virgin coconut oil
6 drops neroli essential oil
4 drops ylang ylang essential oil

1. In a medium bowl, mix the almond oil with the coconut oil.

2. Stir in the essential oils.

3. Using a hand blender, whisk the mixture for 6 to 10 minutes until it's creamy and has increased in bulk. Transfer the mixture to an 8-ounce jar.

APPLICATION: Smooth 1 teaspoon at a time on dry skin after a bath.

STORAGE: Store the tightly sealed jar in a cool, dark place for up to 12 months.

BASIC BATH SALTS

SCENT: YOUR CHOICE   COST: $–$$

MAKES: 16 (1-OUNCE) TREATMENTS

Bathing in mineral-enriched or perfumed water is one of the oldest forms of hydrotherapy. The practice of adding bath salts to a bath was a way of bringing home the medicinal benefits of soaking at a mineral spring to remove toxins from the body. Adding scent to the water brought a luxury touch to the experience, as well as enhanced relaxation. Experiment with bath-salt blends to achieve different moods.

A CLOSER LOOK

The food coloring dyes readily available in any grocery store are water-based and are perfect for creating pastel shades. If you want a more intense shade, consider using gel food coloring, which has a glycerin and corn syrup base. These are harder to find, though some hobby shops and specialty cooking stores carry them. Be sure to choose FDA-approved colorants and dyes, some of which can be found at www.pvsoap.com or www.fromnaturewithlove.com.

½ cup sea salt
½ cup Epsom salts
½ teaspoon (50 drops) essential oil of choice
Colorant or dye, as needed

1. In a medium bowl, mix together the sea salt and Epsom salts.

2. Stir in the essential oils.

3. Add the colorant one drop at a time until the bath salts become the color you desire.

4. Transfer to a 16-ounce jar.

APPLICATION: Add 1 ounce of bath salts to a hot bath as it runs.

STORAGE: Store the tightly sealed jar in a cool, dark location for up to 12 months.

WINTER WARMING COFFEE BODY SCRUB

SCENT: SPICY/CITRUS   COST: $

MAKES: 1 CUP

Cold weather is hard on dry skin; over-heated indoor air takes its toll as well. If your skin appears or feels dry, or if you can scratch your name in the flaky surface of your forearm, it's time to exfoliate. The sugar crystals in this scrub help to remove dry skin, while the orange essential oil soothes, reduces inflammation, and works with the cinnamon essential oil and the caffeine in the coffee to stimulate blood flow.

FYI

Vegetable glycerin is an inexpensive, slippery, colorless, odorless liquid produced from plant oils like palm and coconut. It is readily found in large health food stores and is available by mail order from Amazon.com.

½ cup granulated sugar
½ cup ground coffee (not used coffee grounds)
½ cup vegetable glycerin
12 drops sweet orange essential oil
10 drops cinnamon leaf essential oil

1. In a medium bowl, mix the granulated sugar and the ground coffee.

2. Stir in the vegetable glycerin and mix well. Then add the essential oils and mix to blend well.

3. Transfer the mixture to a 12-ounce jar.

APPLICATION: Use in the bath or shower as a scrub for flaky, dry skin.

STORAGE: Store the tightly sealed jar in a cool, dark place for up to 2 weeks.

SPICY LIME SALT SCRUB

SCENT: CITRUS/SPICY   COST: $$

MAKES: 1¼ CUPS

This is an exfoliating salt scrub with a scent that should equally appeal to men and women. Keep in mind that citrus essential oils are commonly phototoxic—that is, they can cause the skin to have an inflammatory reaction if exposed to UV light shortly after their application. With the particular amounts noted here, make sure that you use steam-distilled lime essential oil, and not cold-pressed, as the cold-pressed lime essential oil is phototoxic, but the essential oil derived from steam distillation is not. If you purchase or only happen to have cold-pressed lime essential oil, do your best to stay out of direct sunlight for about 12 hours.

1 cup fine sea salt
½ cup carrier oil
8 drops lime essential oil
3 drops black pepper essential oil
3 drops ginger essential oil
1 drop patchouli essential oil

1. In a 16-ounce jar, add the salt and then the carrier oil. Using a wooden spoon, stir the oil and salt together until the salt is moist.

2. Add the essential oils and stir again until all the ingredients are combined.

APPLICATION: Use 1 to 3 tablespoons of the scrub in the shower or bath as an exfoliating body scrub, or 1 to 2 teaspoons as a face scrub.

STORAGE: Store the tightly sealed jar in a cool, dark location for up to 12 months.

TIP
Store this scrub in a zip-top bag if you don't have a mason jar or similar container.

GREEN TEA TONER

SCENT: HERBAL   COST: $

MAKES: 1 CUP

The green tea lends a strong herbal note to this toner. The tea and vinegar serve as astringents to close pores and fight oil, while the thyme essential oil has disinfectant and antiseptic properties to clean and tone skin and complement the fresh scent.

SIMPLE SWAP

You can replace the thyme oil with rosemary oil for the same effects but a different scent.

¾ cup brewed green tea, cooled
¼ cup apple cider vinegar
15 drops thyme essential oil

1. In a medium bowl, combine the tea and vinegar.

2. Add the essential oil and stir to mix well.

3. Transfer the mixture to an 8-ounce spray bottle.

APPLICATION: Spritz on your face after cleansing it thoroughly. Allow the toner to air dry.

STORAGE: Store the tightly sealed spray bottle in the refrigerator for up to 3 months.

EASY WHIPPED MOISTURIZER

SCENT: FLORAL   COST: $

MAKES: 1 CUP

With just two ingredients and six minutes of your time, you can create a lovely moisturizing blend. Use it as a facial moisturizer or a body butter. Geranium essential oil is known for its medicinal properties and has been used in cosmetics since ancient times to moisturize skin and fight wrinkles.

1 cup extra-virgin coconut oil (at room temperature)
6 drops geranium essential oil

1. In a small bowl, combine both ingredients. Using a hand mixer with the whisk attachment, whip the lotion for 6 to 10 minutes.

2. Transfer the mixture to an 8-ounce jar.

APPLICATION: Use your fingertips to smooth a small amount of this lotion onto clean, dry skin.

STORAGE: Store the tightly sealed jar in a cool, dark location for up to 12 months.

CITRUS SERUM FOR COMBINATION SKIN

SCENT: CITRUS COST: $

MAKES: 1 OUNCE

If you have combination skin, it's probably oily in the T-zone (forehead, nose, and chin) and dry on the cheeks. Sweet almond oil is a light carrier oil that moisturizes but won't clog pores. It will keep dry skin moisturized without making it oily.

A CLOSER LOOK

Facial serums are lighter than lotions and creams and are meant to be used in conjunction with moisturizers to hydrate and deliver nutrients to the skin. Serums are applied after cleaning and before moisturizing.

1 ounce sweet almond oil
8 drops sweet orange essential oil
7 drops lemon essential oil

In a 1-ounce bottle with a dropper top, combine all the ingredients and shake to mix well.

APPLICATION: Shake before each use. With your fingertips, pat a small amount onto the skin before moisturizing each night at bedtime.

STORAGE: Store the tightly sealed bottle in a cool, dark location for up to 12 months.

HOT OIL TREATMENT FOR BRITTLE HAIR

SCENT: HERBAL   COST: $

MAKES: 1 TREATMENT

Simply put, hot oil treatments restore moisture to hair. There are many factors that contribute to brittle or dry hair, from environmental toxins to hair coloring. Here the essential oil blends with coconut oil, which both moisturizes and prevents the loss of protein to strengthen hair. The rosemary essential oil complements the coconut oil by stimulating the growth of new hair.

4 tablespoons extra-virgin coconut oil
1 drop rosemary essential oil

1. Microwave the coconut oil in a small glass bowl until it is warm. Time will vary depending on microwave strength. Start with 10 seconds and work up.

2. Stir in the essential oil.

APPLICATION:

1. Massage the oil through the hair and down to the scalp.
2. Cover the head with a shower cap (you can buy disposable ones at a beauty supply store) or a towel.
3. Leave on for at least half an hour, but preferably overnight. (Cover your pillow with a towel so you don't ruin the pillowcase.)
4. Rinse out with warm water and then shampoo as usual.

STORAGE: This is a single-use treatment, and no storage is required.

ROSEMARY AND CEDARWOOD DANDRUFF SHAMPOO

SCENT: WOODY/HERBAL   COST: $

MAKES: 1 CUP

Rosemary and cedarwood essential oils blend well together scent-wise, and they both have astringent and exfoliating properties that fight dandruff. Because liquid castile soap can be drying by itself, the addition of coconut oil helps to moisturize, leaving your hair shiny and manageable.

NOTE

Vegetable glycerin is readily available at drug stores like CVS and big-box stores like Walmart. It costs less than $5 for 8 ounces.

½ cup unscented liquid castile soap

¼ cup vegetable glycerin

¼ cup fractionated coconut oil

12 drops rosemary essential oil

12 drops cedarwood essential oil

In an 8-ounce bottle, combine all the ingredients and shake well to mix.

APPLICATION: Shampoo hair with 1 to 2 tablespoons of the soap daily, massaging it into your scalp with your fingertips.

STORAGE: Store in a tightly sealed bottle in your shower for up to 3 months.

TEA TREE–ORANGE DANDRUFF TREATMENT

SCENT: CITRUS/MEDICINAL/MINTY   COST: $

MAKES: 2 OUNCES

Tea tree essential oil is well known for its antidandruff properties. Here, orange essential oil sweetens the scent of this treatment, keeping it from becoming overly medicinal. The peppermint scent cools the scalp as you massage it, while the sweet almond oil moisturizes and exfoliates, removing the flakes.

DID YOU KNOW?

Scalp massages with honey were once used to treat dandruff.

1½ ounces sweet almond oil

10 drops tea tree essential oil

10 drops peppermint essential oil

20 drops orange essential oil

In a 2-ounce spray bottle, combine all the ingredients and shake to mix well.

APPLICATION:

1. Spray over dry hair, making sure the mixture gets down to the scalp. Use your fingers to massage it into your scalp. (You may have to section off your hair with a comb and clips.)
2. Leave the mixture on overnight. Then rinse out the next morning with just a small amount of shampoo.

STORAGE: Store the tightly sealed bottle in a cool, dark place for up to 12 months.

LAVENDER–ROSEMARY HAIR THICKENING TREATMENT

SCENT: FLORAL/HERBAL   COST: $$

MAKES: 1 TREATMENT

If your hair is thinning, it might be because your scalp isn't getting enough stimulation or oxygen. It could also be due to stress, or other factors such as hormones. While this treatment isn't guaranteed to grow new hair, it can help slow the rate of hair loss so your hair stays thicker. The peppermint essential oil stimulates the scalp while the lavender nourishes and relaxes stress.

SIMPLE SWAP

Some women swear by argan oil for thick, shiny hair. While it is a bit more expensive than coconut oil, try replacing half the coconut oil in this recipe with argan oil.

2 tablespoons extra-virgin coconut oil (more or less, depending on hair length)

3 drops lavender essential oil

3 drops rosemary essential oil

In a small glass or metal bowl, mix all the ingredients using a metal spoon or rod.

APPLICATION:

1. Massage the formula into your hair, using your fingers to also gently massage the scalp.
2. Cover your hair with a towel and allow the conditioner to sit for half an hour.
3. Wash and condition your hair as usual.
4. Use once a week in conjunction with your regular washing and conditioning routine.

STORAGE: This is a single-use treatment and no storage is required.

SCALP-STIMULATING CONDITIONER

SCENT: FLORAL/HERBAL   COST: $

MAKES: 1 TREATMENT

A number of things can cause hair loss. While this treatment most likely won't reverse hair loss and cause new hair to grow once it's gone, it may be able to stimulate your scalp and keep you from losing more hair. This conditioner also has a heady, delicious, and addictive fragrance from the ylang ylang and thyme essential oils, both of which may help combat hair loss.

½ cup extra-virgin coconut oil, melted
5 drops ylang ylang essential oil
5 drops thyme essential oil

In a small metal or glass bowl, combine all the ingredients and mix with a metal spoon or rod.

APPLICATION:

1. Massage onto scalp and comb through hair.
2. Leave on the scalp for 15 minutes before washing and conditioning as usual.
3. Use once per week.

STORAGE: This is a single-use treatment and does not require storage.

A CLOSER LOOK

Poor diet can cause thinning hair. Foods that aid in preventing hair loss include walnuts, spinach, halibut, carrots, bok choy, eggs, and Greek yogurt.

NEROLI REPLENISHING HAND CREAM

SCENT: SPICY/CITRUS   COST: $

MAKES: 3 OUNCES

Neroli essential oil has a light, slightly spicy citrus scent that lends a delightful fragrance to this hand cream. The rich, moisturizing hand cream relies on ingredients like cocoa butter, sweet almond oil, and vitamin E for its nourishing, moisturizing properties.

SIMPLE SWAP

For a tropical, fragrant lotion, swap the neroli with ylang ylang essential oil. Or, try a citrus-infused lotion by using orange or grapefruit essential oils.

½ cup cocoa butter

½ cup beeswax

2 tablespoons sweet almond oil

3 vitamin E capsules

10 drops neroli essential oil

1. Fill a small saucepan with a few inches of water and set it on the stove over low heat. Place a metal or glass bowl over the pan so that it fits well.

2. Add the cocoa butter and beeswax to the bowl and wait until the wax melts. Then stir in the almond oil.

3. Pierce the vitamin E capsules and squeeze the oil into the mix.

4. Remove the bowl from the heat and stir in the neroli essential oil using a metal spoon or glass stirring rod.

5. Transfer the mixture to a 10-ounce bottle or jar, and allow it to cool before putting on the lid.

APPLICATION: Smooth over the front and back of hands 2 or 3 times per day, or as needed.

STORAGE: Store the tightly sealed container in a cool, dry place for up to 12 months.

PEPPERMINT MASSAGE GEL

SCENT: MINTY   COST: $

MAKES: 1 OUNCE

One of the most popular treatments in pedicures is massaging the legs with peppermint-infused gel. This peppermint gel is a perfect pick-me-up for tired legs when you've had a difficult day. It's also cooling and soothing if you are experiencing leg soreness or if you have a sunburn. The aloe vera gel moisturizes skin as well.

SIMPLE SWAP

Replace the peppermint with wintergreen or rosemary essential oils for a slightly different scent.

1 ounce aloe vera gel
6 drops peppermint essential oil

In a 1-ounce jar, combine both ingredients and mix with a metal spoon.

APPLICATION: Massage on legs and feet in an upward motion toward the heart.

STORAGE: Store the tightly sealed jar in a cool, dry place for up to 12 months.

ORANGE-PATCHOULI GARDENING SOAP

SCENT: CITRUS/EARTHY   COST: $

MAKES: APPROXIMATELY 3 BARS

The fragrance of this hand soap has a slightly spicy, earthy, and sweetly citrus tone that is uplifting and delicious, leaving your hands smelling wonderful. The recipe also calls for some type of grit, such as ground walnut shells, poppy seeds, or cornmeal, to help scrub the dirt away. The melt-and-pour base in the recipe is a pre-made soap from which you can create a variety of novelty and scented soaps. Using a woody essential oil like juniper or spruce will give the scent a unisex flavor.

GIFT IT

Wrap a bar of soap in parchment, tie it with raffia, and attach a cute label to make a thoughtful gift for your favorite gardener.

1 pound white melt-and-pour soap base, cut into chunks

8 drops orange essential oil

4 drops patchouli essential oil

5 teaspoons "grit" (cornmeal, poppy seeds, ground almonds, ground walnut shells)

1. Fill a small saucepan half full of water and set it on the stove over medium heat until it boils. Place a metal or glass bowl over the pan so that it fits well.

2. Add the soap base and wait until it melts.

3. Remove the bowl from the heat and stir in the essential oils and the grit.

4. Pour into 3 soap molds and allow the soap to harden.

APPLICATION: Wash your hands with the soap using warm water.

STORAGE: Wrap the bars in parchment and store them in zip-top bags in a cool, dark place for up to 12 months.

HEALING HEELS SALVE

SCENT: FLORAL   COST: $

MAKES: APPROXIMATELY 1 CUP

When your heels are so dry that they have deep cracks in them, they require more than a little bit of pumice in the shower. Heel cracks can also be quite uncomfortable. This intensely restorative salve doubles down on the softening ingredients and maximizes skin health with the antiseptic properties of the essential oils and the deeply healing and moisturizing vitamin E.

3 ounces extra-virgin coconut oil
1 ounce beeswax
1 ounce cocoa butter
3 vitamin E capsules
2 ounces sweet almond oil
5 drops geranium essential oil
5 drops lavender essential oil

1. Fill a small saucepan with a few inches of water and set it on the stove over low heat. Place a metal or glass bowl over the pan so that it fits well.

2. Add the coconut oil, beeswax, and cocoa butter and wait until the wax melts.

3. Pierce the vitamin E capsules and squeeze the oil into the wax mixture.

4. Stir in the sweet almond oil and mix well.

5. Remove the bowl from the heat and add the essential oils, mixing well with a metal spoon or glass stirring rod.

6. Transfer the mixture to an 8-ounce jar, and allow it to cool before putting on the lid.

APPLICATION: Rub the mixture on cracked heels at bedtime, and cover with socks.

STORAGE: Store the tightly sealed jar in a cool, dark place for up to 12 months.

ANTIFUNGAL NAIL TREATMENT

SCENT: MEDICINAL   COST: $

MAKES: 2 OUNCES

Nail fungus is a tenacious condition and often requires the aromatherapy equivalent of a tactical nuke to get rid of it. This essential oil blitz is worth it, however, because the most effective of the over-the-counter treatments for the condition has been linked to liver damage. Tea tree essential oil is an anti-fungal, and generally considered to be one of the few essential oils that can be used without dilution. If the condition persists, try using tea tree essential oil undiluted on the nails.

2 ounces carrier oil
12 drops tea tree essential oil
4 drops clove essential oil
2 drops lemon essential oil

In a 2-ounce bottle, combine all the ingredients and shake to mix well.

APPLICATION: Use a cotton swab to "paint" the affected nails with the mixture, applying twice a day until you see signs of healthy new nail growth below the affected nails. Seek medical attention if the condition persists as the nail grows out.

STORAGE: Store in a tightly sealed container in a cool, dry place for up to 12 months.

A CLOSER LOOK

Fungus infections of the fingernails and toenails may seem like more of an unsightly nuisance than a serious medical problem, but if left untreated, the fungus can open up the body to serious systemic infections. In the case of diabetics, especially those suffering from diabetic neuropathy, a toenail fungus could be a gateway to more severe problems, including possible amputation.

NOURISHING CUTICLE LOTION

SCENT: ORIENTAL   COST: $$

MAKES: 1 TREATMENT

One of the essential components of a salon manicure is the application of a nourishing oil to the fingers and toes just before the application of nail polish. Usually, this oil is just a little bit of undiluted vitamin E oil. This blend contains vitamin E and adds the additional benefits of frankincense essential oil to soften and nourish the cuticles.

1 teaspoon vitamin E oil
1 drop frankincense essential oil

In the palm of your hand, mix both the ingredients with a clean finger.

APPLICATION: Massage the blend into the cuticles of each finger and/or toe.

STORAGE: This is a single-use treatment, so no storage is required.

A CLOSER LOOK

Frankincense is great for strengthening brittle nails and also good for nourishing skin. The oil is pricey but this recipe only uses a drop at a time so a very small bottle will last a while.

LAVENDER–ROSEHIP FACE OIL

SCENT: FLORAL   COST: $$

MAKES: 1 OUNCE

Often called "the curse of the Celts" because Europeans of Celtic descent are the most likely ethnic group to suffer from the condition, rosacea is chronic inflammation of the skin. It is most commonly diagnosed between the ages of 30 and 50, and can result in redness, swelling, and irritation of the face. Lavender and chamomile essential oils can help calm breakouts with their gentle anti-inflammatory action. To boost the anti-inflammatory properties of the blend, add a drop of any of the following oils: borage, evening primrose oil, rosewood essential oil, or sea buck-thorn oil.

1 ounce rosehip oil
3 drops lavender essential oil
3 drops chamomile essential oil

In a 1-ounce bottle, combine all the ingredients and shake to mix well.

APPLICATION: Shake before each use. Smooth a few drops on your face at bedtime before using your regular moisturizer.

STORAGE: Store the tightly sealed bottle in the refrigerator for up to 3 months.

DID YOU KNOW?

Prince William has rosacea, as did his mother, Princess Diana. Former president Bill Clinton also has it, as do actresses Cameron Diaz, Renée Zellweger, singer Mariah Carey, and comedian Rosie O'Donnell.

ROSACEA TREATMENT FOR MATURE SKIN

SCENT: CITRUS   COST: $$

MAKES: 1 OUNCE

Rosacea can become more pronounced with age, and what began as a healthy-looking flush to the cheeks as a teen can turn into something far more serious, including disfigurement. This blend uses jojoba oil, which is recommended for use with rosacea. The carrot seed oil provides vitamin A, which is good for aging skin. The bergamot and lavender oils soothe and reduce inflammation.

1 ounce jojoba oil
2 drops carrot seed oil
2 drops bergamot essential oil
2 drops lavender essential oil

In a 1-ounce bottle, combine all the ingredients and shake to mix well.

APPLICATION: Shake before each use. Smooth a few drops onto a clean, dry face once per day.

STORAGE: Store in a tightly sealed container in a cool, dark place for up to 12 months.

POST-PREGNANCY STRETCH MARK SLATHER

SCENT: ORIENTAL/CITRUS   COST: $$

MAKES: ½ CUP

Although this rich body butter is effective in erasing stretch marks due to the vitamin E content, it should not be used as a tummy rub while pregnant because of the myrrh, which can induce premature labor or even miscarriage. Use only after you have delivered your baby to minimize the appearance of stretch marks.

SIMPLE SWAP

To make the butter safe for pregnant women and nursing moms, use frankincense instead of myrrh. Like myrrh, frankincense is a resinous, fragrant essential oil, and though pricey, it's very effective at scar and mark reduction.

2 tablespoons extra-virgin coconut oil

2 tablespoons cocoa butter

2 tablespoons shea butter

1 tablespoon sweet almond oil

3 drops vitamin E oil

8 drops neroli essential oil

6 drops myrrh essential oil

2 drops patchouli essential oil

1. Fill a small saucepan with a few inches of water and set it on the stove over low heat. Place a metal or glass bowl over the pan so that it fits well.

2. Add the coconut oil, cocoa and shea butters, sweet almond oil, and vitamin E to the bowl, whisking constantly as the butters melt.

3. Remove the bowl from the heat and stir in the essential oils using a metal spoon or glass stirring rod.

4. Let the mixture cool, then smooth the body butter into a 4-ounce jar or tin.

APPLICATION: Gently smooth 1 or 2 tablespoons of the lotion onto stretch marks a few times per week.

STORAGE: Store the tightly sealed container in a cool, dark place for up to 12 months.

ANTI-STRETCH MARK BELLY RUB

SCENT: ORIENTAL/MEDICINAL   COST: $$$

MAKES: APPROXIMATELY 1½ CUPS

You can use this lotion to prevent stretch marks during pregnancy, but only after you have completed your first trimester. While there is some controversy over whether it's safe to use essential oils during pregnancy at all, most medical authorities agree that if your pregnancy is trouble-free, it's okay to use gentle essential oils in small amounts. If you have any concerns or questions, consult a licensed aroma-therapist before use.

1 ounce fractionated coconut oil
4 drops vitamin E oil
5 drops lavender essential oil
5 drops frankincense essential oil

In a 2-ounce bottle, combine all the ingredients and shake to mix well.

APPLICATION: Shake before each use. Gently massage 1 to 4 teaspoons of the oil onto the belly, thighs, and arms twice daily.

STORAGE: Store the tightly sealed bottle in a cool, dry place for up to 12 months.

A CLOSER LOOK

Aromatherapy recipes for healing scars and stretch marks often contain Helichrysum (*Helichrysum italicum*) as an ingredient. The essential oil is very expensive (half an ounce, even on sale, costs about $125) but it is well-known as a cicatrizant, meaning it promotes the healing of scars and wounds. If you have any of the oil around, add a couple of drops to the mixture to further enrich the massage rub.

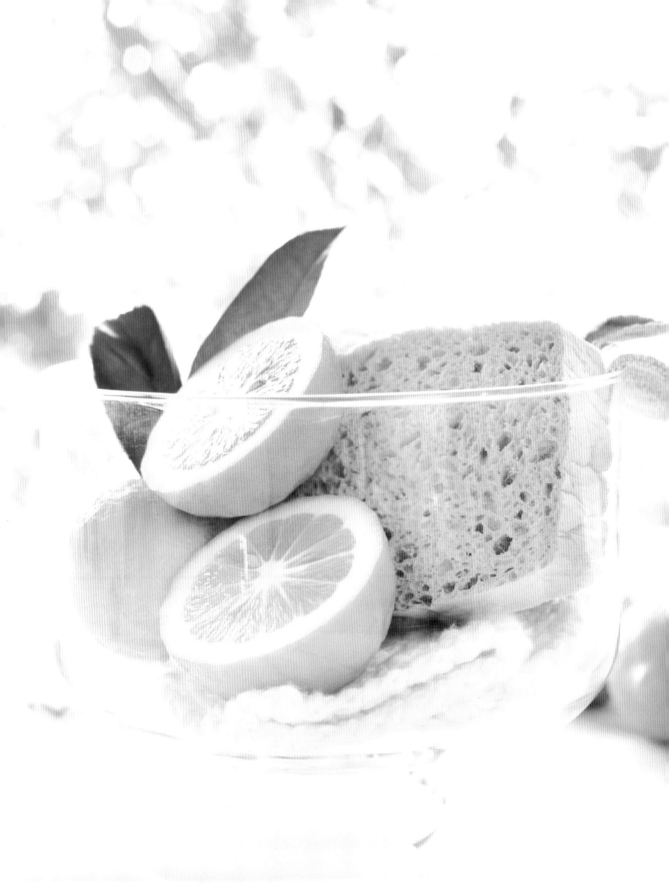

7

REMEDIES FOR THE HOME

Air freshener and deodorizer 194 All-purpose cleaner 196 Kitchen cleaner 197

Bathtub and shower cleaner 198 Toilet cleaner 200 Carpet cleaner 202

Laundry 204 Drains, Panes, and Automobiles 208

Insect Repellent 211 Garden Sprays 216 Pets 218

Just a few generations ago, household cleaning products were a lot more eco-friendly. Scouring powders made from tallow and finely ground quartz had been on the market since the 19th century, but many homemakers still relied on the gentle abrasive power of baking soda to degrease stove tops and scrub away bathtub rings. White vinegar diluted in water served as a glass cleaner, while solutions of pine oil in water were used for mopping floors. In fact, the smell of pine became so associated with the concept of a clean house that companies began manufacturing commercial cleaners with pine fragrance as a selling point. In this chapter you'll find easy DIY recipes for making your own nontoxic, affordable products.

CITRUS CHEER DIFFUSER BLEND

SCENT: CITRUS   COST: $

MAKES: 1 APPLICATION

This is the perfect blend of cheering citrus for use on a rainy day to sweeten the air and lighten your mood. Citrus has a sunny scent that is the perfect, light home fragrance. You can play around with the various citrus oils. For example, try mandarin (tangerine) or petitgrain in place of the bergamot.

2 drops orange essential oil
2 drops bergamot essential oil
2 drops lemon essential oil

In a small glass bowl or bottle, mix together all the ingredients and use as directed in your diffuser.

APPLICATION: Use in a diffuser as directed by the diffuser manufacturer.

STORAGE: This is a single-use product that requires no storage.

SIMPLE SWAP

To make a blend that will sharpen your focus and ability to concentrate, combine 2 drops peppermint, 2 drops cinnamon, and 2 drops tea tree oil.

SIMPLE CITRUS AIR FRESHENER

SCENT: CITRUS   COST: $

MAKES: 1 CUP

This citrus air freshener is the DIY version of popular store-bought brands that contain aerosolized essential oils and not much else despite their price tags. It is quite affordable to make, especially since you can use the cheapest vodka you can find. Feel free to substitute any citrus essential oil you wish.

1 cup distilled water
2 tablespoons unflavored vodka
10 drops lime essential oil

In an 8-ounce spray bottle, combine all the ingredients and shake to mix well.

APPLICATION: Shake before each use. Spritz in the air as needed.

STORAGE: Store the tightly sealed spray bottle in a cool, dark place for up to 12 months.

A CLOSER LOOK

In a widely quoted study conducted by Israeli neurobiologists, scientists discovered "Five Things That Smell Good to Nearly Everyone." The first two scents on the list were lime and grapefruit, followed by bergamot, sweet orange, and peppermint. At the bottom of the list? Musk and patchouli.

THIEVES' OIL ALL-PURPOSE CLEANER

SCENT: MEDICINAL   COST: $

MAKES: 1 PINT

This is a variant of the fabled "Thieves' Oil" that purportedly protected thieves from catching the plague during the Middle Ages. Research shows that the Thieves' Oil blend boosts immunity, and this cleaner has a number of disinfectant essential oils in it. The vinegar cleans without leaving streaks, and any vinegar scent dissipates quickly as it evaporates.

1 cup white vinegar

1 cup distilled water

13 drops lemon essential oil

12 drops clove essential oil

8 drops cinnamon essential oil

8 drops rosemary essential oil

7 drops eucalyptus essential oil

In a 1-pint spray bottle, add the vinegar and water, and then the essential oils. Shake to mix well.

APPLICATION: Shake before each use. Spray on dirty surfaces and wipe off with a damp rag.

STORAGE: Store the bottle in a cool, dark place for up to 12 months.

KITCHEN GREASE-BUSTING CLEANER

SCENT: CITRUS COST: $

MAKES: 1 PINT

When it comes to keeping a clean house, kitchens are as challenging as bathrooms, especially around the stove. If you've cooked up a pound of bacon, you know the kind of sticky film it can leave on the stove top, the nearby counters, the venting hood, and pretty much any other surface within smelling distance. This cleaner harnesses the natural degreasing power of citrus and pure castile soap for a nontoxic product that costs just a fraction of the commercial cleaners available.

NOTE

Baking powder is a mild abrasive that can also be used on its own to clean sinks and countertops. Sprinkle on and use with a wet sponge. The baking powder acts like scouring powder, but without the harsh chemicals.

2 cups distilled water

2 tablespoons baking soda

1 tablespoon unscented liquid castile soap

20 drops lemon essential oil (or other citrus essential oil)

In a 1-pint spray bottle, combine all the ingredients and shake to mix well.

APPLICATION: Shake before using. Spray on greasy surfaces and wipe away with a damp cloth. Leave tougher grease spots in contact with the cleaner for a minute or two before wiping it away.

STORAGE: Store the tightly sealed bottle in a cool, dark spot for up to 12 months.

BATHTUB RING BANISHER

SCENT: MINTY   COST: $

MAKES: APPROXIMATELY 1 CUP

This recipe makes a substance that can also be used on its own to clean sinks and countertops. Sprinkle on and use a wet sponge to gently scour the tub. The washing soda and baking soda scour, and the essential oils disinfect and also leave a fresh aroma. You can easily substitute any other aromatic, disinfectant oil blend.

½ cup baking soda
½ cup washing soda
½ cup liquid castile soap
20 drops tea tree essential oil
12 drops lemon essential oil
10 drops peppermint essential oil

1. In a large bowl, combine the baking soda, the washing soda, and the soap and mix well.

2. Add the essential oils and mix well. Then transfer to an 8-ounce jar.

APPLICATION: Spread 1 to 2 teaspoons of the cleanser on a damp sponge and scrub away at the bathtub ring.

STORAGE: Store the airtight jar in a cool, dark place for up to 12 months.

DID YOU KNOW?

During World War I, American humorist H.L. Mencken wrote an article for the *New York Evening Mail* called "The Neglected Anniversary," a tongue-in-cheek chronicle of the bathtub's history in America. Mencken had meant the story to be a light-hearted bit of fluff to balance the horrible war news filling the papers, but to his surprise, his completely bogus story went viral, in an early-20th-century fashion, with people quoting and requoting it as fact for the rest of the century. His story famously became known as the "Bathtub Hoax."

AFTER-WORKOUT ANTIFUNGAL SPRAY

SCENT: SPICY   COST: $

MAKES: 2 OUNCES

If you regularly hit the gym to work out, chances are you often shower before you return home. If you do, you might want to carry a little bottle of this anti-fungal, antibacterial oil with you and spray it on surfaces where you step with bare feet. The cinnamon essential oil will nuke any fungus spores that might be lurking about, while the alcohol will sanitize surfaces.

1 ounce distilled water
1 ounce rubbing alcohol
8 drops cinnamon bark essential oil

In a 2-ounce spray bottle, combine all the ingredients and shake to blend.

APPLICATION: Shake well before each use. Spray on nonporous surfaces you might touch with your bare feet.

STORAGE: Store the tightly sealed spray bottle in a cool, dark location for up to 12 months.

SIMPLE SWAP

You can replace the cinnamon bark essential oil with tea tree essential oil.

FIZZY TEA TREE TOILET CLEANER

SCENT: MEDICINAL   COST: $

MAKES: 1 APPLICATION

If you ever made a baking soda and vinegar volcano in an elementary science class, you have seen the chemical reaction that occurs when you mix baking soda (a base) with vinegar (an acid). That chemical reaction, combined with the de-germing properties of tea tree essential oil, will leave your toilet smelling fresh. You can easily replace the tea tree essential oil with eucalyptus essential oil.

10 drops tea tree essential oil
½ cup baking soda
½ cup white vinegar

1. In a small bowl, combine the tea tree essential oil and the baking soda.

2. Dump the scented baking soda directly into the toilet bowl.

3. Immediately add the vinegar to the toilet bowl.

APPLICATION: When the mixture begins to foam, scrub the toilet with a toilet brush. Flush when finished cleaning.

STORAGE: This is a single-use application so no storage is required.

DID YOU KNOW?

The crescent moon–shaped odor venting hole seen in most cartoon images of outhouses dates from the earliest use of these outdoor toilets. Two different shapes once marked which gender could use the privies: star-shaped venting holes for the men and crescent moon–shaped holes for the women. For some reason historians can't explain, more women's outhouses have survived.

CITRUS-VINEGAR DISINFECTANT SPRAY

SCENT: CITRUS   COST: $

MAKES: 1 PINT

This citrus-infused vinegar toilet deodorizer and disinfectant is a nice alternative to either pine-scented or the more medicinal tea tree/rosemary/eucalyptus concoctions. It is made with one of the cheapest essential oils available and leaves behind a nice, happy citrus scent in your bathroom.

1 cup white vinegar
6 drops lemon essential oil
4 drops tea tree essential oil

In an 8-ounce spray bottle, add the vinegar and then the essential oils. Shake to blend well.

APPLICATION: Shake well before each use. Spray on the surfaces you want to disinfect and wipe away with a damp cloth.

STORAGE: Store the tightly sealed spray bottle in a cool, dark place for up to 12 months.

CARPET SPOT REMOVER FOR SYNTHETIC FIBERS

SCENT: HERBAL   COST: $

MAKES: 3 CUPS

If you have a wet vacuum or steam carpet cleaner, use this spot remover in place of plain water or a commercial store-bought cleaner. This blend works for carpets with synthetic fibers. Do not use it on carpet with natural fibers.

DID YOU KNOW?

Rosemary has a long history as a carpet cleaner. In medieval times when the floors of manor houses were covered by carpets of rushes that were not changed more than every year or so, "strewing herbs" were sprinkled on the floor to scent the air. The most commonly used strewing herbs were lavender, mint, sage, oregano, marjoram, and rosemary.

1 cup white vinegar

2 cups water

40 drops (⅓ teaspoon) rosemary essential oil

1. In a 16-ounce spray bottle, combine the vinegar and water, and shake to mix well.

2. Add the rosemary essential oil and shake again to mix all the ingredients.

APPLICATION: Shake well before using. Spray on the spot you want to remove from the carpet until it is saturated. Using a white cloth, dab at the spot to lift it. Once it's gone, spray the spot again and use a wet vac or steam cleaner to go over the area.

STORAGE: Store the tightly sealed spray bottle in a cool, dark place for up to 12 months.

NATURAL SPOT REMOVER FOR NATURAL FIBER CARPETS

SCENT: MINTY   COST: $

MAKES: 1 CUP

This minty spray combines peppermint essential oil and liquid dish soap to tackle spots on natural fiber carpets. Be sure when you clean the carpet you dab at the spot. Don't rub it, which can make the spot set in. If you remove the liquid dish soap, you can also use this minty spray as a general air freshener.

1 cup water
1 teaspoon biodegradable liquid dish soap
2 drops peppermint essential oil

1. In an 8-ounce spray bottle, combine the water and soap, and shake to mix well.

2. Add the essential oil and shake again to mix all the ingredients.

APPLICATION: Shake before each use. Spray on the spot until it is completely wet. Allow the remover to sit for 5 minutes. With a clean white towel, dab at the spot until it is gone. Reapply as needed.

STORAGE: Store the tightly sealed spray bottle in a cool, dark place for up to 12 months.

HOMEMADE DRYER SHEETS

SCENT: MEDICINAL   COST: $$

MAKES: 12 REUSABLE DRYER SHEETS

These homemade dryer sheets not only re-purpose those orphan socks that everyone has but also provide a safe, nontoxic alternative to the chemical-laden commercial products that cost more. The dryer sheets smell good, they prevent static cling for items coming out of the dryer, and you can use them multiple times. Likewise, the vinegar softens the fabric, and it doesn't leave behind a vinegary scent.

SIMPLE SWAP

These leave clothing very lightly scented. If you prefer a different scent, feel free to play with other essential oils and blends to find one that pleases you.

6 mismatched shin-length socks
½ cup white vinegar
8 drops tea tree essential oil
3 drops lavender essential oil

1. Cut open the socks vertically, spreading them out like a butterfly. Then cut the socks up the center to make 2 equal-sized strips each, for a total of 12 strips.

2. In a small mixing bowl, add the vinegar and essential oils, and mix well.

3. Drizzle the mixture over the fabric strips, making sure each piece is evenly saturated. Don't squeeze off any excess liquid—it'll be absorbed by your new dryer sheets.

APPLICATION: Use one sheet in the dryer per load of laundry. To reuse the sheets, return them to the container with the other unused sheets that still contain the vinegar solution. When the sheets no longer hold a scent, mix up another batch and drizzle it over the sheets in the container.

STORAGE: Store the sheets together in an airtight container.

DIY LAUNDRY STAIN REMOVER

SCENT: CITRUS   COST: $

MAKES: ¾ CUP

This simple recipe works as well as commercial spray-on stain removers, but without their toxic skin and eye irritants. If the stain is particularly stubborn, add a few tablespoons of the blend to some baking soda and rub the paste into the fabric using an old toothbrush. The lemon essential oil in the mixture will go to work on the stain right away. For very stubborn stains, you can even use the lemon essential oil directly on the spot.

½ cup nontoxic liquid soap

¼ cup hydrogen peroxide

100 drops (approximately 1 teaspoon) lemon essential oil

In a 4-ounce spray bottle, add the soap and the hydrogen peroxide, then add the essential oil and shake to mix.

APPLICATION: Spritz onto the stain to saturate it. Using a white cotton cloth, agitate the spot, or scrub with a toothbrush for stubborn set-in stains. Rinse the article and then wash as usual.

STORAGE: Store the spray bottle in a cool, dark location for up to 12 months.

OLD-FASHIONED LAUNDRY DETERGENT

SCENT: MEDICINAL   COST: $

MAKES: 2 CUPS

This detergent is especially good for washing baby clothes, as it does not contain dyes or other harsh chemicals that can linger on fabrics and cause irritation and allergic reactions. The tea tree oil fights germs, but if you don't like the scent you can replace it with any other scent, such as lavender or lemon.

1 cup borax
1 cup washing soda
½ cup grated bar soap
20 drops tea tree essential oil

In a 1-quart mason jar, combine all the ingredients and stir with a metal fork or spoon to mix well.

A CLOSER LOOK

Before there were spray-on stain removers for laundry, there was washing soda, which is also known as "sodium carbonate." You can find Arm & Hammer brand washing soda (the same people who sell baking soda) in the laundry detergent section of any large supermarket. Or you can make your own washing soda: 1) Set the oven to 400°F. 2) Spread a box of baking soda on the bottom of a metal cookie sheet or a rectangular glass baking pan. 3) Bake for an hour, stirring the baking soda about halfway through. The heat releases carbon dioxide and the end result will be grainier and more yellowish than baking soda.

APPLICATION: Use ¼ to ½ cup in your laundry, washing as usual.

STORAGE: Store in a tightly sealed jar in your laundry room.

LINEN WATER

SCENT: FLORAL   COST: $$

MAKES: 2 CUPS

Before the invention of steam irons, clothing had to be dampened before ironing so that the hot metal would press out the wrinkles more efficiently. Traditionally, lavender petals or essential oil is the ingredient used to fragrance linen water, but any scent that pleases you can be used for fresh-smelling clothes after you iron them.

SIMPLE SWAP

For a subtle rose scent, substitute geranium or palmarosa for the lavender or mix the two for a lovely French garden scent.

2 cups distilled water
2 tablespoons vodka
25 drops lavender essential oil

1. In a 16-ounce spray bottle, add the water and vodka, and shake to blend.

2. Add the lavender essential oil and shake to blend again.

APPLICATION: Shake before using. Mist clothing lightly before ironing.

STORAGE: Store the tightly sealed spray bottle in a cool, dark location.

CITRUS DRAIN FLUSH

SCENT: CITRUS   COST: $

MAKES: 1 DRAIN TREATMENT

No matter how clean you keep your kitchen, bad smells can sometimes originate in the garbage disposal, trash compactor, or garbage can. You can always take out the trash and wash out a garbage bin, but if a bad smell is wafting from your sink's drain hole you need to treat it at the source. One quick way to kill the odor, at least temporarily, is to cut up a lemon or lime and run it through the garbage disposal. A longer-lasting remedy is this Citrus Drain Flush. The flush will both kill the smell and help avoid a buildup of gunk that could clog up your sink.

2 gallons water
1 cup baking soda
300 drops (1 tablespoon) lemon essential oil
1 cup white vinegar

1. In a large stockpot over high heat, bring the water to a boil.

2. In a medium metal or glass dish, mix together the baking soda and essential oil.

APPLICATION:

1. Slowly pour half the boiling water (1 gallon) down the noxious-smelling drain, and return the rest to the stove to continue boiling.
2. Pour the baking soda mix down the drain.
3. Pour the white vinegar down the drain.
4. Allow the vinegar–baking soda interaction to work for 5 minutes, then flush the drain with the remainder of the boiling water.

STORAGE: This is a single-use treatment so no storage is required.

DIY GLASS CLEANER

SCENT: MEDICINAL   COST: $

MAKES: 1½ CUPS

Although glass-making technology has been known since Roman times, up until the late 19th century only the wealthy could afford glass windows. (The poor made do with window-coverings made of oiled hide, slices of mica, parchment, or even simple shutters.) This DIY Glass Cleaner contains nothing but ingredients that would have been known to the 19th-century homemaker, and it makes windows sparkle without streaks.

SIMPLE SWAP

For a fresh citrus scent, replace the tea tree essential oil with any of the citrus essential oils, such as grapefruit, lemon, or mandarin.

2 cups warm water
2 tablespoons cornstarch
¼ cup rubbing alcohol
¼ cup white vinegar
10 drops tea tree essential oil

1. In a medium bowl filled with warm water, dissolve the cornstarch, stirring to make sure there aren't any lumps.

2. Stir in the rubbing alcohol and vinegar.

3. Using a funnel, transfer the liquid to a 16-ounce spray bottle.

4. Add the essential oil and shake to blend.

APPLICATION: Shake before using. Spray the cleaner on glass surfaces and wipe off with a clean cloth such as a microfiber towel, which won't leave streaks.

STORAGE: Store the tightly sealed spray bottle in a cool, dark place for up to 12 months.

TEA TREE ANTI-MOLD SPRAY

SCENT: MEDICINAL   COST: $

MAKES: 1 QUART

Mold is more of a problem in humid climates, but it thrives in enclosed environments. Most garages don't have windows, and garage doors are rarely left open for any length of time, so the environment stays fetid. Mold is an opportunistic organism—it grows on concrete floors, metal shelving, and wooden rafters. You can find it inside washers and dryers, growing on plastic garbage cans, and even in piles of recycling stored between trash pickups. This spray can help fight mold in your garage—or anywhere else it grows. The tee tree essential oil's antifungal properties will kill the mold spores. Other essential oils with antifungal properties include cedarwood, cilantro, clary sage, clove, lavender, lemon, and rosemary.

4 cups distilled water
400 drops (4 teaspoons) tea tree essential oil

In a 16-ounce spray bottle, combine all the ingredients and shake to mix.

APPLICATION: Shake well before using. Spray the mixture in damp areas to inhibit mold growth, and spray on moldy surfaces. Leave in contact with the surface for 1 hour before wiping clean with a rag.

STORAGE: Store the tightly sealed spray bottle in a cool, dry location for up to 12 months.

DID YOU KNOW?

In the wake of the devastating floods caused by Hurricane Katrina and Hurricane Sandy, mold production soared in the affected areas causing a variety of respiratory illnesses and other allergic reactions. Public health officials warned that mycotoxins released by the mold spores could be mutagenic (causing damage to genes) as well as trigger neurological damage.

CITRONELLA–PEPPERMINT MOSQUITO REPELLENT

SCENT: CITRUS/MINTY   COST: $

MAKES: 4 OUNCES

Citronella is a well-known insect repellent, and it is common in a number of commercial insect repellent products. It has a lemony scent that bugs, particularly mosquitos, avoid. Likewise, it is free of some of the scary chemicals, such as DEET, that are in commercial mosquito repellents.

WARNING

Peppermint is not safe to use on children 6 years old or younger. For a child-safe bug option, see Lea Harris's Bug Bite Soother recipe on page 32.

2 ounces distilled water

1½ ounces witch hazel

1 teaspoon carrier oil

35 drops citronella essential oil

35 drops peppermint essential oil

In a 4-ounce spray bottle, combine all the ingredients and shake to mix well.

APPLICATION: Shake before each use. Spray the repellent on the body before going outdoors. Allow it to absorb into skin before putting clothes on.

STORAGE: Store the tightly sealed spray bottle in a cool, dry place for up to 12 months.

ROLL-ON GERANIUM BUG REPELLENT

SCENT: FLORAL/CITRUS   COST: $

MAKES: 1 OUNCE

Wear this bug repellent whenever you're headed somewhere notorious for bugs and mosquitos. The scent of geranium essential oil is known to repel gnats, mosquitoes, and ticks. It has a pleasant scent, so you won't smell like you're wearing bug spray, and the coconut oil will smooth and condition your skin.

1 ounce fractionated coconut oil
6 drops geranium essential oil

In a 1-ounce glass bottle with a roller top, combine all the ingredients. Shake to mix.

APPLICATION: Roll the oil onto pulse points. Reapply as necessary.

STORAGE: Store the tightly sealed roller bottle in a cool, dark place for up to 12 months.

ROACH SPRAY

SCENT: MINTY/MEDICINAL   COST: $$

MAKES: ½ CUP

Roach infestations can be frustrating because they are so difficult to resolve. A popular belief is that roaches are so indestructible they'll survive a nuclear explosion. That may be so, but hit them with this homemade 1-2-3 punch of essential oils and they won't want to stick around long enough to find out. This DIY spray is much safer than commercial roach sprays, and contains cypress and peppermint essential oils, scents that roaches find unpleasant and avoid.

1 tablespoon salt
½ cup water
10 drops tea tree essential oil
10 drops peppermint essential oil
5 drops cypress essential oil

1. In a small bowl, dissolve the salt in the water.

2. Pour the salt water into an 8-ounce spray bottle, and add the essential oils. Shake to mix well.

APPLICATION: Spray the solution in areas where roaches are visible, as well as any cracks or crevices where they might lurk. Spray twice a day, shaking the mixture before each use.

STORAGE: Store the tightly sealed spray bottle in a cool, dark place for up to 12 months.

NOTE

Another DIY roach-killing concoction can be made by combining 1 cup borax with ⅓ cup granulated sugar and sprinkling the mixture where roaches congregate. It works fine by itself, but adding a few drops of peppermint essential oil makes it smell nice and gives it a scent that repels the roaches.

SIMPLE SPIDER SPRAY

SCENT: MINTY   COST: $

MAKES: 1 CUP

Spiders hate strong scents, and peppermint is one of the most noxious to them. For even more potent protection against invading arachnids, use the peppermint oil without dilution to wipe down window sills, doorjambs, and anywhere else they might be gaining entry to your home.

1 cup distilled water
12 drops peppermint essential oil

In a 12-ounce spray bottle, add the water and then the essential oil. Shake well.

APPLICATION: Shake well before each use. Spray the solution in areas where spiders may gain entry into your home.

STORAGE: Store the tightly sealed spray bottle in a cool, dark place for up to 12 months.

DID YOU KNOW?

In China, farmers deliberately attract spiders to their cotton fields to eat the boll weevils that would otherwise destroy their crops.

DUST MITE DETERRENT

SCENT: MEDICINAL/MINTY   COST: $$

MAKES: 1 TREATMENT

Dust mites can collect in areas such as mattresses and pillows, where they may trigger allergies, asthma, and other respiratory issues. This formulation allows you to treat dust mites in mattresses, cushions, and pillows with the antimicrobial properties of lavender and peppermint essential oils. Other scents that repel dust mites include clove, rosemary, and wintergreen.

A CLOSER LOOK

According to WebMD, 20 million Americans are allergic to dust mites and have symptoms ranging from red, watery, itchy eyes to swollen and stuffed noses. Dust mite allergies peak in the summer, particularly in humid weather, so keeping bedding clean (washing in water hotter than 130°F and drying in a hot dryer) and treating mattresses with a deterrent may be necessary to remove the tenacious infestations.

1 cup baking soda
5 drops lavender essential oil
5 drops peppermint essential oil

1. In an 8-ounce mason jar, add the baking soda and then the essential oils.

2. Stir with a metal fork to make sure that there are no clumps in the baking soda and that the essential oils are distributed evenly.

APPLICATION:

1. Strip the bed and wash the bed linens.
2. If you have a baking sifter, pour the scented baking soda into it and sift the mixture all over the top of the bare mattress. Otherwise, pour the mixture into a mesh strainer and use that to shake the powder across the mattress.
3. Let the mixture sit for at least an hour before vacuuming off.
4. Make the bed with clean sheets.
5. Repeat once a month or as necessary.

STORAGE: Store the tightly sealed jar in a cool, dark place for up to 12 months.

NONTOXIC WEED KILLER

SCENT: SPICY   COST: $

MAKES: 1 QUART

Some gardeners swear that all you need to get rid of garden weeds is a good dose of boiling water. While that might be effective, it is impractical to carry a tub of boiling water around with you as you garden. This spray works the same way those noxious chemical sprays do to kill weeds, and it won't leave dangerous chemical residues.

DID YOU KNOW?

Herbal weed-killer remedies have been in use since classical times, but they co-existed for centuries with remedies based on folk magic and supernatural lore. Hanging a mare's skull in the garden was said to protect against caterpillar infestation, for instance, and burying a toad in a field of millet was another agricultural charm against pests, both botanical and zoological.

1 quart white vinegar
¼ cup salt
1 teaspoon biodegradable liquid dish soap
400 drops (4 teaspoons) clove essential oil

1. In a large bowl, mix together the vinegar, salt, and dish soap.

2. Add the essential oil and mix well.

3. Using a funnel, transfer the mixture to a 16-ounce spray bottle.

APPLICATION: Spray solution directly on the weeds you wish to kill.

STORAGE: Store the tightly sealed spray bottle in a cool, dark place for up to 12 months.

PEPPER SPRAY FOR PLANT PESTS

SCENT: SPICY   COST: $

MAKES: 1 QUART

The same essential ingredient in pepper sprays used for self-defense (capsicum) has a long history in aromatherapy, from use as an ingredient in analgesic creams to relieve arthritis pain to its use as a pest-repellent for garden plants. Spraying plants with this spicy concoction won't harm them, but it will keep insects from turning your garden into a salad bar.

1 quart water
1 teaspoon biodegradable liquid dish soap
100 drops (1 teaspoon) black pepper essential oil

In a 16-ounce spray bottle, add the water and dish soap and then add the essential oil. Shake to mix well.

APPLICATION: Shake well before using and spray on plants to repel bugs.

STORAGE: Store the tightly sealed spray bottle in a cool, dark location for up to 12 months.

A CLOSER LOOK

Using hot pepper as a bug repellent will not affect the taste of any vegetables you grow, because the plant won't absorb the essential oil.

NIX TICKS BLEND FOR DOGS

SCENT: FLORAL   COST: $$

MAKES: 2 OUNCES

Just as geranium oil can repel pests for humans, it also does so for dogs. This gentle, safe remedy will keep your dog tick-free, and you use such a small amount that it is perfectly safe. It's a great way to protect your dog without all the harsh and potentially neurotoxic chemicals in commercially available flea and tick preparations.

A CLOSER LOOK

In addition to its many other qualities, geranium oil is valued for its antistress properties. The oil is also helpful in treating eczema and moisturizing dry skin, which is just as important for dogs as humans.

2 ounces water

3 to 6 drops geranium bourbon essential oil

In a 2-ounce bottle with a spray top, combine the ingredients and shake vigorously to blend.

APPLICATION: Shake well before using. Spritz your dog at the base of the tail and at the back of the neck before going for a walk or sending him out into the yard.

STORAGE: Store the capped bottle in a cool, dark place for up to 12 months.

CALMING SPRAY FOR DOGS

SCENT: EARTHY/FLORAL   COST: $$

MAKES: ½ CUP

If you have a dog that suffers from anxiety, this spray can be a game-changer. Whether your dog gets anxious during thunderstorms, nervous when you leave the house, or upset when you have guests, the lavender and vetiver will calm her down. You can also use this calming spray for easily excited dogs.

½ cup distilled water
6 drops lavender essential oil
6 drops vetiver essential oil

In a 4-ounce spray bottle, add the water and then the essential oils. Shake vigorously to blend.

APPLICATION: Shake well before using. Lightly mist the mixture on the dog's bedding. *Do not* spray directly on the animal.

STORAGE: Store the tightly sealed spray bottle in a cool, dark place for up to 12 months.

DID YOU KNOW?

A lot of anecdotal evidence suggests aromatherapy with vetiver essential oil blends might help kids with ADHD. While clinical evidence is lacking, parents who prefer not to go the Ritalin route are quietly recounting their experiences with vetiver, lavender, and other relaxing essential oils in the treatment of their children.

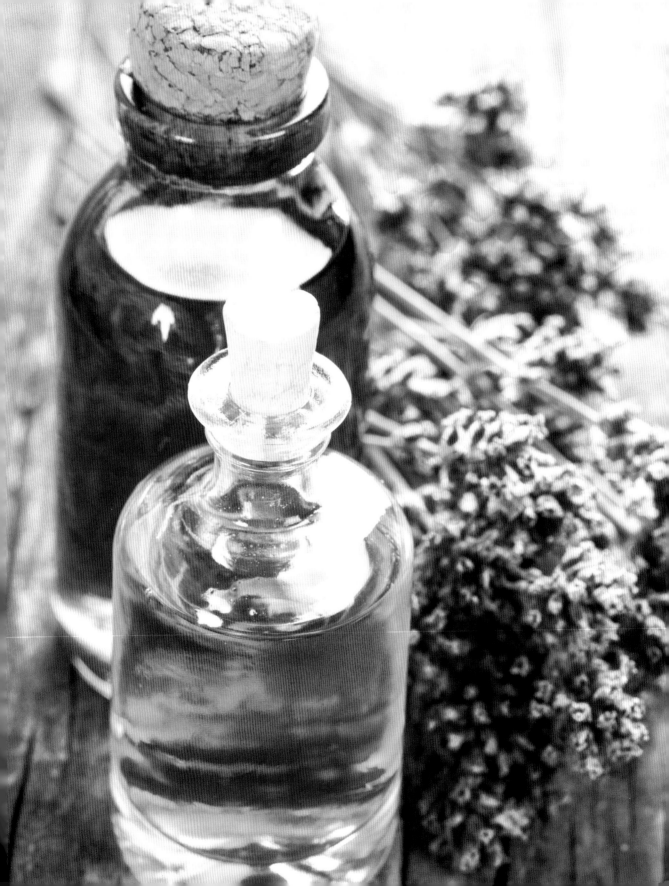

8

PERFUME RECIPES

Eau de Parfum 222 Eau de Toilette 224 Eau de Cologne 226 Splashes 228

Perfumery is an ancient art dating back at least 4,000 years that began as something akin to alchemy. As with winemaking, a specialized language has evolved around perfume production, from the terminology used to describe a perfume's creator to the ways we discuss how a scent evolves on the skin.

Eau de parfum is the most concentrated form of a fragrance blend—a little bit goes a long way.

Eau de toilette is a more diluted, and thus weaker, fragrance formulation than eau de parfum.

Eau de cologne, or simply "cologne," is the most diluted form of perfume sold, and typically refers to a man's fragrance.

The term *splash* originally referred to any astringent, healing liquid applied (splashed on) after shaving to heal and tighten the skin.

A NIGHT IN MARRAKESH SOLID PERFUME

SCENT: ORIENTAL   COST: $$$

MAKES: 3 OUNCES

Because this sensuous blend contains benzoin, you shouldn't use it while you are pregnant. The perfume has a deep base resin note from benzoin with a floral middle and top note coming from the lush fragrance of ylang ylang. The result is a dark, mysterious aroma in a lovely, solid perfume. If you prefer, you can replace the benzoin with a few drops of frankincense essential oil.

GIFT IT

Small solid perfumes make great stocking stuffers as well as party favors. Craft stores carry perfume lockets and rings designed to be filled with the solidified fragrance. Look for them anywhere jewelry findings are sold.

3 tablespoons beeswax
3 tablespoons coconut oil
6 drops benzoin essential oil
6 drops ylang ylang essential oil

1. Fill a small saucepan with a few inches of water and set it on the stove over low heat. Place a metal or glass bowl over the pan so that it fits well.

2. Add the beeswax to the bowl and wait until it melts. Then stir in the coconut oil and whisk until melted.

3. Remove the bowl from the heat and add the essential oils.

4. Immediately transfer the mixture into a 3-ounce jar or tin, and allow it to cool and harden before putting on the lid.

APPLICATION: Rub a small amount of the perfume onto pulse points.

STORAGE: Store the tightly sealed container in a cool, dark place for up to 12 months.

FLEUR CLASSIQUE PARFUM

SCENT: FLORAL/CITRUS   COST: $$

MAKES: 4 OUNCES

If you love florals, this is the perfect fragrance for you. The heady perfume blend combines sweet ylang ylang essential oil with citrus and other florals to create a sophisticated, layered scent that isn't too heavy. The vodka will help preserve and extend the fragrance, and it won't smell like you spilled a drink on yourself when you applied your perfume.

SIMPLE SWAP

Winter grapefruit or lemon essential oils will also work well in place of the orange in this blend. Blood orange is pricier, but gives the scent a whole new character.

½ cup carrier oil

2 tablespoons unflavored vodka

15 drops ylang ylang essential oil

6 drops lavender essential oil

3 drops bitter orange essential oil

1. In an 8-ounce atomizer bottle, add the carrier oil and vodka, and shake to blend.

2. Add the essential oils and shake to blend all the ingredients.

APPLICATION: Spritz lightly on pulse points, or spray lightly in the air and walk through the fragrance cloud.

STORAGE: Store in the tightly sealed atomizer in a cool, dark place for up to 12 months.

GARDEN IN THE WOODS EAU DE TOILETTE

SCENT: WOODY/FLORAL   COST: $$

MAKES: 16 OUNCES

Amyris essential oil has a woody scent reminiscent of sandalwood and is often referred to as West Indian sandalwood. It is a less expensive option if you enjoy the scent of sandalwood but not the price. This light floral scent will transport you to a lovely woodland garden with its soothing aroma. If you happen to have sandalwood on hand, use it in place of the amyris.

DID YOU KNOW?

One of the oldest toilet water formulations still in use is "Carmelite water," a concoction based on lemon balm and spices that was originally crafted by Carmelite nuns in the 14th century.

2 cups distilled water

4 tablespoons unflavored vodka

10 drops geranium essential oil

10 drops bergamot essential oil

5 drops amyris essential oil

1. In a 16-ounce spray bottle, add the water and vodka and shake to blend.

2. Add the essential oils and shake again to mix all the ingredients.

APPLICATION: Spritz onto pulse points.

STORAGE: Store in the spray bottle in a cool, dark place for up to 12 months.

LAVENDER–LEMON EAU DE TOILETTE

SCENT: FLORAL/CITRUS   COST: $$

MAKES: 1 OUNCE

Floral and citrus combine well, and this light scent won't overpower. Lemon and lavender create a classic combination that smells clean and fresh, perfect for a summer afternoon or a casual event. Dab it on your pulse points, and the light scent will surround you as you go about your day.

GIFT IT

Tiny bottles of this light fragrance make very nice bridesmaid gifts, or work well as part of a "goodie bag" at a bridal or baby shower.

1 ounce unflavored vodka

2 tablespoons distilled water

5 drops lavender essential oil

5 drops lemon essential oil

1. In a 1-ounce bottle, add the vodka and water, and shake to mix.

2. Add the essential oils and shake again to mix.

3. Allow the perfume to mellow for 24 hours before using.

APPLICATION: Shake before each use. Dab on pulse points.

STORAGE: Store the tightly sealed bottle in a cool, dark place for up to 12 months.

WINTER SPICE COLOGNE

SCENT: WOODY/MINTY   COST: $$

MAKES: 2 OUNCES

Traditionally, heavier perfumes are worn in winter, but this light fragrance will remind the wearer of an evergreen forest dusted with snow. With cypress, pine, and peppermint, it's the perfect holiday fragrance, either to wear yourself or give as a gift. The scent works well for women and men.

2 ounces unflavored vodka

3 drops cypress essential oil

2 drops pine essential oil

2 drops black pepper essential oil

2 drops peppermint essential oil

1 drop cardamom essential oil

In a 2-ounce bottle, combine all the ingredients, and shake to blend.

APPLICATION: Shake before each use. Dab on pulse points.

STORAGE: Store the tightly sealed bottle in a cool, dark place away from vibration.

HUNGARY WATER

SCENT: CITRUS/FLORAL   COST: $$

MAKES: 8 OUNCES

This summery cologne is based on the fabled "Hungary Water" formula first crafted for Queen Elizabeth of Hungary in the 14th century. The light, citrus formula with floral mid notes and earthy bottom notes may boost mood. With such an intoxicating scent, it's a cologne fit for a queen.

1 cup unflavored vodka

30 to 35 drops bergamot essential oil

½ teaspoon lavender essential oil

¼ teaspoon neroli essential oil

1. In a 4-ounce bottle with an atomizer lid, combine all the ingredients, and shake well to blend.

2. Store the mixture in the refrigerator for a week to mellow before using.

DID YOU KNOW?

The Queen of Hungary is not the only monarch in history whose name has had a signature scent. Recipes exist for Cleopatra's beeswax and rose face cream and sea salt and cream scrub. Queen Elizabeth I favored a scent composed of musk and Damask rose water, according to a 400-year-old recipe for the fragrance. Pierre-François Pascal Guerlain (of the perfume house that still bears his name) created Eau de Cologne Impériale for Emperor Napoleon III and his wife Empress Eugénie, and also crafted custom scents for Queen Victoria. Franco-Russian perfumer Beaux (the "nose" who created No. 5 for Chanel) created a now-lost fragrance inspired by Catherine the Great, who also inspired a fragrance known as "The Empress' Favorite Bouquet."

APPLICATION: Shake before using. Spritz a little cologne on pulse points, or spray some in the air and walk through the mist.

STORAGE: Store the tightly sealed bottle in a cool, dark place for up to 12 months.

UNISEX CITRUS & SPICE SPLASH

SCENT: CITRUS/SPICY   COST: $$

MAKES: 1 OUNCE

Citrus and spice scent combinations have long proved favorites with both men and women. This unisex blend of grapefruit and ginger is uplifting and energizing, so it's perfect to splash on after your morning shave and/or shower. The fragrance will linger without overpowering.

SIMPLE SWAP

Lemon, wild orange, or lime essential oil work well in this splash in place of the grapefruit.

1 ounce unflavored vodka
2 drops grapefruit essential oil
2 drops ginger essential oil
2 drops vetiver essential oil

In a 1-ounce bottle, combine all the ingredients, and shake to blend.

APPLICATION: Shake before each use. Splash 1 teaspoon of the blend on the face and as desired on the body, avoiding the eyes.

STORAGE: Store the tightly sealed bottle in the refrigerator for up to 12 months.

HEALING AFTERSHAVE SPLASH

SCENT: WOODY   COST: $$

MAKES: 1 OUNCE

This healing aftershave splash refreshes as it soothes irritated skin. The scents of cedarwood, cypress, and bergamot essential oils are distinctly masculine with a lovely woody character. Store it in the refrigerator so it cools even more.

1 ounce unflavored vodka
2 drops cedarwood essential oil
2 drops cypress essential oil
2 drops bergamot essential oil

In a 1-ounce bottle, combine all the ingredients, and shake to blend.

DID YOU KNOW?

Cedarwood has long been prized for its fragrance. It was used ceremonially by the Egyptians as part of the mummification process, and was burned by the Greeks and Romans in classical times to sweeten the air. In modern perfumery it is often used as a base note and lends its distinctive fragrance to scents such as Black Cashmere by Donna Karan and Cèdre by Parfums 06130.

APPLICATION: Shake before each use. Splash a teaspoon or so of the aftershave on the face after shaving, avoiding the eyes.

STORAGE: Store the tightly sealed bottle in the refrigerator for up to 3 months.

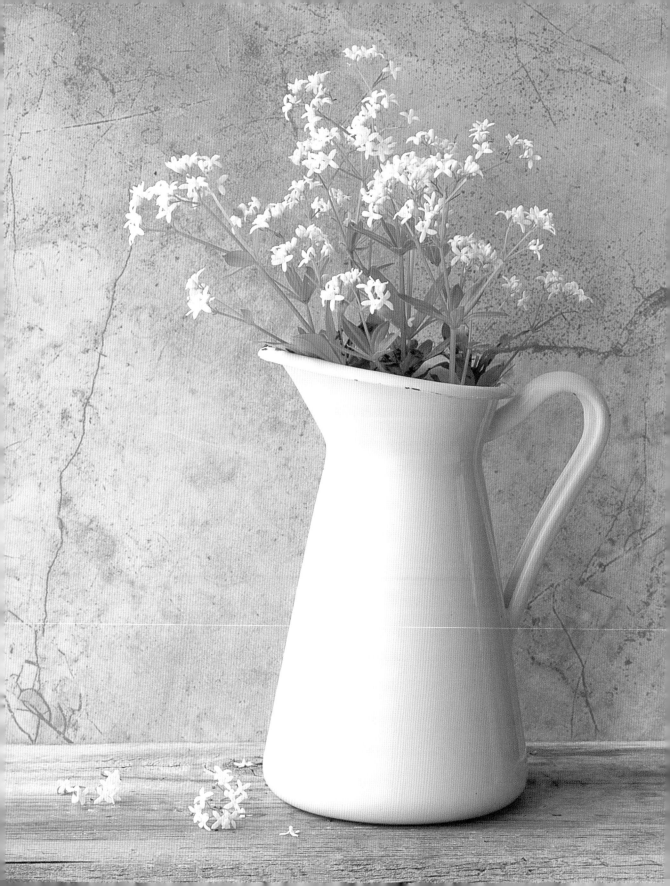

MEASUREMENT CONVERSIONS

VOLUME EQUIVALENTS (LIQUID)

US STANDARD	US STANDARD (OUNCES)	METRIC (APPROXIMATE)
2 tablespoons	1 fl. oz.	30 mL
¼ cup	2 fl. oz.	60 mL
½ cup	4 fl. oz.	120 mL
1 cup	8 fl. oz.	240 mL
1½ cups	12 fl. oz.	355 mL
2 cups or 1 pint	16 fl. oz.	475 mL
4 cups or 1 quart	32 fl. oz.	1 L
1 gallon	128 fl. oz.	4 L

OVEN TEMPERATURES

FAHRENHEIT (F)	CELSIUS (C) (APPROXIMATE)
250°F	120°C
300°F	150°C
325°F	165°C
350°F	180°C
375°F	190°C
400°F	200°C
425°F	220°C
450°F	230°C

VOLUME EQUIVALENTS (DRY)

US STANDARD	METRIC (APPROXIMATE)
⅛ teaspoon	0.5 mL
¼ teaspoon	1 mL
½ teaspoon	2 mL
¾ teaspoon	4 mL
1 teaspoon	5 mL
1 tablespoon	15 mL
¼ cup	59 mL
⅓ cup	79 mL
½ cup	118 mL
⅔ cup	156 mL
¾ cup	177 mL
1 cup	235 mL
2 cups or 1 pint	475 mL
3 cups	700 mL
4 cups or 1 quart	1 L

WEIGHT EQUIVALENTS

US STANDARD	METRIC (APPROXIMATE)
½ ounce	15 g
1 ounce	30 g
2 ounces	60 g
4 ounces	115 g
8 ounces	225 g
12 ounces	340 g
16 ounces or 1 pound	455 g

GLOSSARY

ABSOLUTE: An alcohol-based essential oil extracted using a solvent. It contains essential oil compounds but differs from distilled essential oils. Many flower fragrances are absolutes rather than essential oils.

ADULTERATED: An oil that contains anything but pure, 100-percent essential oil, or one that has been blended with another pure essential oil from another plant.

ANALGESIC: A substance that relieves pain. Eucalyptus, lavender, and rosemary have analgesic properties.

ANIMALIC: A term used in perfumery to describe a musky, animal-like scent. While these scents were formerly harvested from animals like the civet, nowadays the "note" is almost always synthetic.

ANTIPRURITIC: A substance that stops itching, such as witch hazel or basil essential oil.

BULKING: Using plants from the same species but from different harvests to bring down the cost of a specific oil.

CARMINATIVE: A substance that prevents gas from forming in the intestinal tract.

CHOLAGOGUE: A substance that stimulates the flow of bile from the liver, which aids in digestion. Rosemary has this property.

CICATRIZANT: A substance that promotes the healing of wounds and scars. Tea tree oil is a powerful cicatrizant.

EMOLLIENT: A substance that softens and smooths skin by adding moisture. Coconut and jojoba oils are emollients. Peppermint has emollient properties.

FEBRIFUGE: Something that reduces a fever. Peppermint oil is a febrifuge.

FRACTIONATED: A fraction of the original substance. This book's recipes occasionally call for fractionated coconut oil. The process of fractioning removes the less-stable triglycerides from coconut oil, leaving a more saturated oil that, as a result, is more stable.

HUMECTANT: A substance that attracts and binds moisture to the skin. Glycerin and honey are both humectants.

INDOLIC: A nice way of saying that a perfume has a fecal scent. It's well known that a number of flowers, most particularly jasmine, have a fecal quality to their aroma, and for some, when that note develops as a perfume ("opens"), the smell can be quite nasty. On the other hand, there are indolic notes in some of the most famous perfumes ever created, including *Joy* by Jean Patou, *No. 5* by Chanel, and *Olene* by Diptych.

INSOLUBLE: A substance that is not capable of being dissolved in liquid such as water.

NEAT: Undiluted. Opinion varies widely on whether any essential oils are suitable for applying to the skin neat. No recipe in this book calls for the neat application of any essential oil.

PHOTOTOXIC: Substances that magnify skin sensitivity to the sun, increasing the possibility of sunburn or other damage. All cold-pressed citrus oils are phototoxic.

SENSITIZATION: A reaction similar to an allergic reaction that may occur when essential oils build up in the system, or when someone applies an undiluted essential oil directly on the skin. You can avoid sensitization by following dilution guidelines exactly and giving your body a break from oils occasionally. If you do have a sensitization reaction to a certain essential oil, you need to avoid that oil in the future.

THERMOGENIC: A substance that creates heat through metabolic stimulation. Black pepper and cinnamon are thermogenic and often used in "warming" lotions and pain-relief creams.

VERMIFUGE: A substance that destroys and/or expels parasitic worms. Essential oils with vermifuge properties include bergamot, lavender, rosemary, and tea tree.

QUICK REFERENCE GUIDE TO AROMAS AND OILS

CITRUS

Bergamot
Citronella
Grapefruit (all varieties)
Lemon
Lemongrass
Lime (all varieties)
Mandarin (Tangerine)
Melissa
Neroli
Orange (all varieties)
Petitgrain
Yuzu

EARTHY

Anise
Bay
Clary sage
Fennel
Oakmoss
Patchouli
Sage
Vetiver

FLORAL

Calendula
Chamomile
Geranium
Helichrysum
Jasmine
Lavender
Palmarosa
Rose
Ylang ylang

HERBACEOUS/HERBAL/GREEN

Basil
Bay
Chamomile
Fennel
Lavender
Marjoram
Oregano
Parsley
Rosemary
Sage
Thyme
Yarrow

MEDICINAL

Cajeput
Eucalyptus
Niaouli
Tea tree
Wintergreen

MINTY

Basil
Peppermint
Spearmint
Wintergreen

ORIENTAL

Frankincense
Myrrh
Patchouli
Sandalwood

SPICY

Bay
Black pepper
Cardamom
Celery
Cinnamon (all varieties)

WOODY

Amyris
Cedarwood
Clove
Coriander
Cumin
Cypress
Fir needle
Frankincense
Ginger
Juniper
Nutmeg
Oak
Oakmoss
Pimento
Pine (all varieties)
Rosewood
Sandalwood
Spruce
Vetiver

RESOURCES

BLOGS

Almost Makes Perfect
www.almostmakesperfect.com
This is DIY with loads of style. Especially good as inspiration for gift projects.

Crunchy Betty
www.crunchybetty.com
Offers home remedies, natural beauty recipes, and directions for making nontoxic cleaners.

Growing Up Herbal
www.growingupherbal.com
A blog dedicated to raising children naturally, GUH is full of tips for dealing with childhood ailments using essential oils, herbs, and other natural remedies.

Herbal Riot
herbalriot.tumblr.com
An intriguing site that offers insight into traditional and magical uses of herbs and essential oils. There are also recipes for herbal remedies and entertaining historical background factoids.

Scratch Mommy
www.scratchmommy.com
Theme: "Life, from scratch." Tons of ideas and directions for DIY projects, especially homemade cosmetics.

Wellness Mama
www. wellnessmama.com
Theme: "Simple answers for healthier families." DIY with mobile apps, a podcast, books, and tons of ideas for healthy things you can make yourself.

BOOKS

Essential Oils Natural Remedies: The Complete A–Z Reference of Essential Oils for Health and Healing. Berkeley, CA: Althea Press, 2015.

Jones, Marlene. *The Complete Guide to Creating Oils, Soaps, Creams, and Herbal Gels for Your Mind and Body.* Ocala, FL: Atlantic Publishing Group, Inc., 2010.

Lea, Sandra. *The Encyclopedia of Candlemaking Techniques: A Step-by-Step Visual Guide.* Philadelphia, PA: Running Press, 1999.

Purchon, Nerys and Lora Cantele. *The Complete Aromatherapy and Essential Oils Handbook for Everyday Wellness.* Toronto: Robert Rose, Inc., 2014.

Siegler-Maier, Karyn. *The Naturally Clean Home: 100 Safe and Easy Herbal Formulas for Nontoxic Cleansers.* N. Adams, MA: Storey Publishing, 1999.

ESSENTIAL OILS BRANDS

Aura Cacia
www.auracacia.com
The site doesn't just offer essential oils for sale; it provides recipes for their use—easy DIY projects for the bath, the home, kids, pets, and more.

Eden Botanicals

www.edenbotanicals.com

Eden Botanicals carries the rare Yuzu essential oil in a variety of sizes, from a 20–30 sampler ($2) to a 1 kg. package that costs nearly $1,000.

Esoteric Oils

www.essentialoils.co.za

This company is interested in educating their customers in the history and use of essential oils as well as selling them on their no-frills website, which is deliberately low-key.

Mountain Rose Herbs

www.mountainroseherbs.com

This friendly site is a great resource for anyone looking for a concise database of essential oil properties.

Plant Therapy

www.planttherapy.com

Plant Therapy carries some of the harder-to-find essential oils, including blood orange, May Chang (aka Litsea Cubeba), and Rosalina.

INGREDIENTS FOR HEALTH, HEALING, COSMETIC CARE, AND THE HOME

BATH SALTS

The main ingredients for bath salts—sea salt, kosher salt, and baking soda—are readily available at any supermarket. Other ingredients that are often added to the mix include Epsom salts (found at any drug store) and rock salt (aka "ice cream salt") and are also readily available. Once you get into ingredients like Dead Sea salt and pink Himalayan salt, however, you'll need to find a company that specializes in the product you want. Some sources:

SaltWorks

www.saltworks.us

A Pacific Northwest company, SaltWorks provides premium-grade specialty salts to the wholesale, retail, and consumer market. Their products are intended for use in both food and personal care products.

San Francisco Salt Company

www.sfsalt.com

Their motto is "Relaxing the world, one bath at a time." They carry dendritic sea salt (said to help bath salt mixtures retain their scent longer), non-scented sea salts, as well as pink Himalayan salt and the more prosaic Epsom salts. They also carry a line of gourmet salts like smoked cherrywood sea salt for cooks who like to season their food with a grain of salt.

BEAUTY BUTTERS

Coconut oil is readily available at any grocery store but ingredients like cocoa butter, lanolin, shea butter, and mango butter may be harder to find locally. The following companies offer these ingredients by mail:

Butters and Bars
www.butters-n-bars.com

From Nature with Love
www.fromnaturewithlove.com

The Herbarie
www.theherbarie.com

Mountain Rose Herbs
www.mountainroseherbs.com

BOTTLES, CONTAINERS & JARS

Abundant Health
www.abundanthealth4u.com
A good source for roll-on bottles.

Ananda Apothecary
www.anandaapothecary.com
A good source for droppers and pipettes, which allow for more precise measuring of your oils.

Best Bottles
www.bestbottles.com
This place is a bottle bonanza. In addition to roll-on bottles in several sizes and in several colors, they also sell atomizer bottles, perfume vials, and apothecary-style jars. They also offer refillable metal shell atomizer bottles. They sell their bottles by the piece and can also accommodate wholesale orders.

Bottles and Foamers
www.bottlesandfoamers.com
This site is excellent if you are searching specifically for a foaming-soap dispenser.

Bulk Apothecary
www.bulkapothecary.com

The Container Store
www.containerstore.com
In addition to offering all sorts of boxes and storage options, the Container Store has a lot of cute containers for gifting your DIY products. (Or, you can just browse their catalogue and get ideas for doing it yourself.)

Etsy
www.etsy.com
Once a site devoted solely to handmade arts and crafts, Etsy is now a source for all things DIY. Many of the artisans offer supplies like essential and fragrance oils, candle waxes, and soap-making ingredients along with the products they made themselves.

General Bottle Supply
www.bottlesetc.com
This West coast company, established in 1926, is a wholesale distributor of a wide variety of glass bottles, plastic containers, and assorted caps. They offer both amber and blue aromatherapy bottles as well as droppers and mister, shaker, and pump caps. Because they are a distributor, however, the smallest amount of each item that can be ordered is 48 pieces.

SKS Bottle & Packaging
www.sks-bottle.com
Plastic, glass, and metal containers for all your aromatherapy needs. Bottles with a wide array of tops (brush tops, spray tops, screw-on tops) are available. Available sizes range from 5 mL to 100 mL.

CANDLEMAKING

CANDLE DYE

It's hard to find organic, natural dyes for candles. Dyes come in meltable color blocks, liquid, and chips. You should avoid the chips if you want to go all natural as most are made with paraffin. You can find "Liquid Eco-friendly" candle dye at:

Ruhl Bee Supply
www.ruhlbeesupply.com
While primarily a source for those interested in beekeeping—they supply everything from "hive kits" to starter sets of actual bees—Ruhl Bee Supply also sells natural candlemaking and soap-making supplies including essential oils.

BEESWAX

Brushy Mountain Bee Farm
www.brushymountainbeefarm.com
In addition to providing beeswax for candlemaking, Brushy Mountain provides all-natural ingredients for DIY cosmetics, soap, and honey mead and wine.

CANDLE WICKS

It's important to use candle wicks that don't contain lead cores. A candle with a lead-core wick releases five times the amount of lead considered hazardous for children and exceeds EPA pollution standards for outdoor air, according to the Consumer Product Safety Commission (CPSC), which banned lead wicks in 2003. Metal cores in American-made wicks contain zinc.

Wicks coming from other countries may contain lead, though, so here's a test to check: Rub a piece of white paper over the top of an unburnt wick. If a pencil-like mark is left behind, the wick has lead; if it doesn't leave a mark, it doesn't have lead.

Some sources of candle wicks are:

Candlescience
www.candlescience.com
The site features candlemaking help, FAQs, and video tutorials on how to do everything from choose the right size wick to DIY recipes for sea shell candles and specialty fragrance blends.

Jo-Ann
www.joann.com
The ubiquitous brick-and-mortar craft store also has an online presence selling general craft and candlemaking supplies as well as fabric.

Lone Star Candle Supply
www.lonestarcandlesupply.com
Their site features candlemaking tutorials as well as a useful trouble-shooting FAQ. They also sell digital scales for weighing wax, thermometers, and pouring pots to make the process easier.

COSMETIC CLAY

Used for making facial and body masks, in soaps and scrubs, and also for wraps and packs. Any clay you use for your DIY projects should be "cosmetic-grade" clay. Different clays contain different nutrients, and although all have detoxifying properties, some are more effective than others.

From Nature With Love

www.fromnaturewithlove.com

The company has been in business since 1997, and sells natural and conventional ingredients for cosmetics and other aromatherapy products. They have an extensive DIY recipe database, including instructions for making four kinds of soap (cold-process, hand-milled, hot-processed, and melt-and-pour).

The Original Soap Dish

www.thesoapdish.com

In addition to cosmetic-grade clay, they sell various salts, fragrances, fruit powders, and dried herbs. They also offer a wide range of candle-, soap-, and lotion-making supplies, including glycerin. For crafters interested in giving their products as gifts or venturing into a home business, they offer eco-packaging options.

SOAP MAKING

Melt-and-pour soap base for "cold-press" soap is widely available at craft stores like Michael's and Hobby Lobby. "Cold-press" is the easiest method for making DIY soap, and a great first step for those interested in making soaps scented with essential oils.

Bramble Berry Soap Making Supplies

www.BrambleBerry.com

Bulk Apothecary

www.BulkApothecary.com

The Chemistry Store

www.ChemistryStore.com

WEBSITES

Amazon

www.amazon.com

If you're interested in one-stop shopping, this online mega-retailer is the place to start. They provide access to the brands you'd buy anyway, and the reviews and ratings can help you decide which brand choices are the best. If you prefer a more personalized experience, here are some other sources to consider.

AromaWeb

www.aromaweb.com

This site bills itself as "Your source for aromatherapy and essential oil information" and it does not disappoint. It's a clearinghouse for information, a database for DIY recipes, a link hub for more information, and more, more, more.

Easy Aromatherapy Recipes

www.easy-aromatherapy-recipes.com

This site is a great place to start if you're looking for inspiration for making your own products with essential oils. The site is filled with easy DIY recipes for health, beauty, and home cleaning. There are also lots of tips for gift ideas.

Homemade Mommy

www.homemademommy.net

Theme: "Keeping it real in a fake food world." Real food recipes, DIY recipes for cosmetics, and home remedies using essential oils.

Joelle's Sacred Grove

www.joellessacredgrove.com

For those interested in the sacred and magical meanings of herbs and oils, this site offers a lot of lore.

Learning about EOs

www.learningabouteos.com

Recipes, safety information, resources—even giveaways. Site owner Lea Harris encourages interaction with her readers, and has a thriving social media presence as well.

National Association for Holistic Aromatherapy

www.naha.org

Primarily focused on professional education for the practicing or aspiring aromatherapist, this site also serves as a clearinghouse for information on sustainability issues, and offers a calendar of upcoming aromatherapy events and how-tos like "How to find an aromatherapist."

The Online Herbal Encyclopedia

www.cloverleaffarmherbs.com

This is an organized source for more information about the properties of individual plants and their essential oils. Filled with little bits of lore and factoids specific to the herbs, which make the herbal profiles entertaining reading.

Pinterest

www.pinterest.com

Free to join, this social media site is filled with step-by-step instructions for all kinds of DIY projects, including thousands of recipes for DIY aromatherapy projects.

Your Aromatherapy Guide

www.your-aromatherapy-guide.com

Maintained by Jan Randall, a holistic therapist born in Cornwall and transplanted to France, this site offers tips for baby and pet aromatherapy as well as basic information about essential and carrier oils. For those interested in some of the more esoteric edges of aromatherapy practice, she also has sections on astrology and chakras.

REFERENCES

BOOKS

Althea Press. *Essential Oils for Beginners: the Guide to Get Started with Essential Oils and Aromatherapy*. Berkeley, CA: Althea Press, 2013.

Cunningham, Scott. *The Complete Book of Incense, Oils & Brews*. Woodbury, MN: Llewellyn Publications, 2014.

Kelville, Kathi and Mindy Green. *Aromatherapy: A Complete Guide to the Healing Art, Second Edition*. Berkeley, CA: Crossing Press, 2009.

Largo, Michael. *The Big, Bad Book of Botany: The World's Most Fascinating Flora*. New York, NY: William Morrow Paperbacks, 2014.

Laws, Bill. *Fifty Plants that Changed the Course of History*. Ontario, Canada: Firefly Books, 2011.

Life Science Publishing. *Essential Oils Pocket Reference, Sixth Edition*. Lehi, UT: Life Science Publishing, 2014.

Miller, Light, and Bryan Miller. *Ayurveda & Aromatherapy*. Delhi, India: Motilal Banarsidass, 1998.

Perchon, Nerys and Lora Cantele. *The Complete Aromatherapy and Essential Oils Handbook for Everyday Wellness*. Ontario, Canada: Robert Rose, 2014.

Pollan, Michael. *The Botany of Desire: A Plant's Eye View of the World*. New York, NY: Random House, 2002.

Rupp, Rebecca. *How Carrots Won the Trojan War: Curious (but True) Stories of Common Vegetables*. N. Adams, MA: Storey Publishing, 2011.

Schiller, Carol and David Schiller. *500 Formulas for Aromatherapy*. New York, NY: Sterling Publishing Co., 1994.

Stewart, Amy. *The Drunken Botanist: The Plants That Create the World's Great Drinks*. New York, NY: Workman Publishing Co., 2013.

Stewart, Amy. *Wicked Plants: The Weed That Killed Abraham Lincoln's Mother and Other Botanical Atrocities*. New York, NY: Algonquin Books, 2009.

Tourles, Stephanie L. *Hands-On Healing Remedies*. N. Adams, MA: Storey Publishing, 2012.

Worwood, Valerie Ann. *The Complete Book of Essential Oils & Aromatherapy*. Novato, CA: New World Library, 1991.

Zhi-Shui, Li. *The Private Life of Chairman Mao*. New York, NY: Random House, 1996.

PAPERS/WEBSITES

"Aromatherapy and Essential Oils." Accessed June 3, 2015. www.ncbi.nlm.nih.gov/pubmedhealth/PMH0032645/.

Ballard, Clive G., John T. O'Brien, Katharina Reichelt, and Elaine K. Perry. "Aromatherapy as a Safe and Effective Treatment for the Management of Agitation in Severe Dementia." *The Journal of Clinical Psychiatry* 63.7 (2002): 553–58.

Flaxman, D. and P. Griffiths. "Is Tea Tree Oil Effective at Eradicating MRSA Colonization? A Review." Br J Community Nurs. 10(3): 123-6. PubMed NCBI. Accessed May 8, 2015: www.ncbi.nlm.nih.gov/pubmed/15824699.

Howdyshell C. "Complementary Therapy: Aromatherapy with Massage for Geriatric and Hospice Care—a Call for an Holistic Approach." PubMed News. Accessed May 12, 2015. www.ncbi.nlm.nih.gov/pubmed/9677958.

Jepson R. G., Williams G., Craig J.C. "Cranberries for Preventing Urinary Tract Infections." Cochrane (2013). www.cochrane.org /CD001321/RENAL_cranberries-for-preventing-urinary-tract-infections.

Mercola, Joseph. "Herbal Oil: Comfrey Oil Benefits and Uses." Mercola.com. Accessed June 3, 2015. articles.mercola.com/herbal-oils /comfrey-oil.aspx.

Moss, Mark, and Lorraine Oliver. "Plasma 1,8 Cineole Correlates with Cognitive Performance Following Exposure to Rosemary Essential Aroma." *Therapeutic Advances in Psychopharmacology* 2.3 (2012): 103–113.

National Association for Holistic Aromatherapy. What Are Essential Oils? NAHA, Accessed June 3, 2015. www.naha.org/explore -aromatherapy/about-aromatherapy /what-is-aromatherapy.

National Association for Holistic Aromatherapy. What Is Aromatherapy? NAHA, Accessed June 3, 2015. www.naha.org/explore-aromatherapy /about-aromatherapy/what-are-essential-oils.

National Association for Holistic Aromatherapy. Safety NAHA, Accessed June 3, 2015. www.naha.org/explore-aromatherapy/ about-aromatherapy/safety.

PLOS Computational Biology. "Predicting Odor Pleasantness with an Electronic Nose." Accessed May 2, 2015.journals.plos.org /ploscompbiol/article?id=10.1371/journal .pcbi.1000740.

Redwood, Daniel. "Interviews with People Who Make a Difference: Alternative and Complementary Medicine: Interview with Marc Micozzi, MD." 1995. Healthy.Net. www.healthy.net/scr/interview.aspx?Id=239

University of Maryland Medical Center. "Lavender." Last modified January, 1, 2015: http://umm.edu/health/medical/altmed /herb/lavender#ixzz3aH5KoHl0.

WebMD. "Understanding Cold Sores Basics." WebMD. Accessed June 3, 2015. www.webmd .com/skin-problems-and-treatments/guide /understanding-cold-sores-basics.

INDEX OF ESSENTIAL OILS

A

amyris, 224

Angelica, 22

aniseed, 22

B

basil, 22, 30, 51, 125, 139

benzoin, 222

bergamot, 30, 52, 90, 92, 134, 141, 145, 147, 148, 155, 156, 163, 189, 194, 224, 227, 229

birch, 22

bitter orange, 223

black pepper, 22, 30, 53, 91, 111, 129, 173, 217, 226

C

cajeput, 30

calendula, 22, 54, 101, 120

camphor, 22

cardamom, 226

cedarwood, 22, 30, 55, 113, 126, 178, 210, 229

chamomile, 30, 56, 120, 121, 147, 151, 155, 156, 157, 188

cilantro, 210

cinnamon, 30, 91, 98, 130, 194, 196

cinnamon bark, 22, 57, 199

cinnamon leaf, 16, 22, 57, 138, 172

citronella, 211

clary sage, 22, 30, 58, 140, 141, 210

clove, 22, 30, 59, 91, 96, 127, 138, 153, 186, 196, 210, 215, 216

comfrey, 105

coriander, 60

cypress, 22, 30, 61, 93, 130, 135, 157, 164, 213, 226, 229

E

eucalyptus, 22, 30, 40, 44, 62, 98, 109, 110, 132, 136, 149, 150, 196, 200

F

fennel, 22, 122, 163

fir needle, 119

frankincense, 30, 63, 130, 135, 164, 187, 191

French lavender, 22

G

geranium, 22, 64, 101, 113, 118, 126, 134, 135, 140, 141, 145, 146, 157, 164, 167, 175, 185, 207, 212, 218, 224

ginger, 30, 65, 91, 129, 143, 173, 228

grapefruit, 30, 66, 117, 147, 156, 209, 228

H

helichrysum, 105, 107, 191

hyssop, 22, 30

J

jasmine, 30, 31

juniper, 22, 67, 104, 117, 127, 144, 147, 184

L

lavender, 30, 40, 43, 44, 68, 90, 92, 93, 95, 99, 100, 106, 108, 114, 119, 121, 126, 132, 134, 135, 136, 137, 138, 139, 146, 147, 150, 153, 155, 156, 166, 180, 185, 188, 189, 191, 202, 204, 207, 210, 215, 219, 223, 225, 227

lemon, 30, 40, 44, 69, 92, 103, 110, 113, 118, 131, 133, 139, 142, 144, 147, 166, 168, 176, 186, 194, 196, 197, 198, 201, 205, 208, 209, 210, 225, 228

lemongrass, 70

lime, 71, 173, 195, 228

M

mandarin, 30, 209

marjoram, 123, 202

Melissa (lemon balm), 14, 30

mint, 202

Mugwort, 22

myrrh, 22, 72, 153, 190

N

neroli, 170, 182, 190, 227

niaouli, 73

nutmeg, 22, 30, 74, 91, 129

O

oakmoss, 22

orange, 30, 31, 75, 89, 91, 112, 136, 143, 172, 179, 184, 194

oregano, 22, 76, 202

P

palmarosa, 77, 118, 145, 147, 207

parsley, 22

patchouli, 30, 78, 119, 173, 184, 190

peppermint, 30, 31, 40, 42, 79, 89, 97, 98, 102, 108, 109, 111, 112, 122, 129, 133, 140, 152, 183, 184, 194, 198, 203, 211, 213, 214, 215, 226

pine, 30, 80, 119, 150, 226

R

rose, 30, 31

rosemary, 14, 22, 30, 81, 98, 106, 108, 110, 115, 123, 139, 150, 157, 162, 178, 180, 182, 196, 202, 210, 215

rosewood, 30

rue, 22

S

sage, 22, 202

sandalwood, 30, 82, 113, 118, 128, 129, 135, 149, 155, 168

Spanish lavender, 22

spearmint, 142

spikenard, 15

spruce, 119, 184

sweet orange, 176

T

tansy, 22

tarragon, 22

tea tree, 24, 30, 31, 40, 44, 83, 93, 94, 96, 97, 98, 102, 103, 104, 115, 116, 124, 126, 131, 134, 136, 137, 138, 139, 150, 154, 157, 158, 159, 179, 186, 194, 198, 200, 201, 204, 206, 209, 210, 213

thyme, 95, 98, 123, 138, 157, 162, 174, 181

V

vetiver, 84, 129, 219, 228

W

wild orange, 228

wintergreen, 22, 30, 215

Y

ylang ylang, 17, 30, 85, 128, 129, 170, 181, 222, 223

INDEX

A

abortifacient, 22

abscesses, 137

absolutes, 19, 232

acne, 162–163

Acorelle, 53

Acqua di Gio, 71

ADHD, 218

adulterated, 232

Adventurer II, 67

aging skin, 164

air freshener and
      deodorizer, 194–195

alcohol-based perfumes, 17

Allen, Maria, 121

allergies
    dust mites, 215
    essential oils, 22

all-purpose cleaner, 196

almond (bitter) essential oil, 24

Alzheimer's disease, 103

AmeriColor food colorings, 171

analgesic, 232

Angel, 78

animal bites, 98

animalic, 232

antipuritic, 232

antiseptic spray, 136

anxiety, 89

apricot kernel oil, 33

argan oil, 33

Armani, 71

Arm & Hammer washing soda, 206

aromapeutics, 17

aromas
    blending essential oils, 24–26
    quick reference guide, 234–235

aromatherapy, 9
    basics, 13–28
    baths, 14
    cost-effectiveness, 26
    depression, 15
    essential oils, 14
    facials, 14
    history, 15, 17
    massages, 14
    multipurpose products, 26
    over-the-counter medicines
        alternatives, 26
    product quality, 27
    products as gifts, 27
    reducing toxic chemicals in
        home, 26
    signature scent, 27
    spa industry, 14
    Western world, 17

aromatherapy blends
    beeswax, 41
    Five Thieves' Disinfectant
        Spray, 44
    Lavender Moisturizing Hand
        Cream, 43
    Lemon-Peppermint Lip
        Balm, 42

aromatherapy mistakes, 45–46

arthritis, 91

artificial scents, 16

astrology, 81

athlete's foot, 93–95

attar of roses, 17

Aurien Nigra, 53

Australia, 82, 83

avocado oil, 33

Ayurvedic medicine, 17, 64, 70, 75

B

babies, 24
    Baby Bum Lotion, 121
    Baby-Safe Salve, 126
    Chamomile-Calendula Diaper
        Cream, 120
    Essential Cradle Cap Oil
        Blend, 113
    essential oils, 24
    Gentle Lavender Oil Blend, 114
    Massage Lotion for Babies, 90
    Old-Fashioned Laundry
        Detergent, 206
    Rosemary-Lavender Salve for
        Bruises, 106

bad breath, 96–97

baking powder, 197

baking soda, 95, 100

balanced fragrances, 24

balsam of Mecca, 72

baths, 14

bath salts
    ingredients, 237
    shopping for supplies, 37

Basic Bath Salts, 171

bathtub and shower cleaner,
    198–199

bayberry, 17

beauty butters ingredients, 238

beauty supply stores, 37

Beaux, 227

bee stings, 100

beeswax, 41, 239

    Basic Lip Balm, 165

    candles, 41

    essential oils and, 146

benzene, 19

Bible, 15

birch bark tonic, 17

bites, 98–99

Black Cashmere, 229

Black Forest, 80

Black Phoenix Alchemy Lab, 80

Black Vetiver, 84

blending essential oils

    aromas, 24–26

    floral aromas, 25

    fragrance notes, 24–26

    herbal aromas, 25

    medicinal aromas, 25

    spicy aromas, 25

    woody aromas, 25

blisters, 101–102

blogs, 236

Boccaccio, 15

body odor, 103–104

boldo essential oil, 24

Bonaparte, Napoleon, 135

brain, 19

brand reputation of essential
    oils, 31

brittle hair, 177

brittle nails, 187

Brosseau, Jean Charles, 85

bruises, 105–106

bug bites

Bug Bite Soother, 32

bug repellent, 217

bulking, 232

burns, 107–108

Butters and Bars, 169

C

cade essential oil, 24

calamus essential oil, 24

Calvin Klein, 67

camphor (brown) essential oil, 24

candle dye, 239

candle makers, 9

candles

    bayberry, 17

    beeswax, 41, 239

    candle dye, 239

    handmade, 27

    ingredients, 239

    PMS Blend Votive Candle, 146

    shopping for supplies, 37

    wicks, 239

Carmelite water, 224

carminative, 232

carpet cleaner, 202–202

carrier oils, 16, 21

    shopping for, 31, 33–35

cassia essential oil, 24

castile soap, 104

castor oil, 34

Caswell-Massey, 71

cedarwood, 229

Cédre, 229

certified essential oils, 31

chamomile hydrosol, 16

Chanel, 232

chapped lips, 165–167

children

    ADHD, 218

    Basic Burn Gel, 107

    essential oils, 24

    Eucalyptus-Mint Rub, 109

    Lavender-Tea Tree Lice
        Treatment, 138

    peppermint essential oil, 211

    Take a Deep Breath Calming
        Diffusion Oil, 89

China, 214

Chinese medicine, 17, 72, 78

cholagogue, 232

Chopard, 75

Ciara, 77

cicatrizant, 232

cinnamon bark essential oil, 16

cinnamon leaf essential oil, 16

citronella, 70

citronella oil, 70

citrus essential oils, 25, 30

CK IN2U for Her, 67

Clarke, Mae, 66

Cleopatra, 164, 227

Clinton, Bill, 188

cloth diapers, 121

Cochrane Collaboration, 154

cocoa butter, 118

coconut oil, 33, 118

CO_2 extraction, 18

cognitive performance, 14

cold pressing. *See* expression

colds, 109–110

cold sores, 102

College of Physicians, 14

combination skin, 176

congestion, 109–110

conjunctivitis, 54

constipation, 111–112

Cook, James, Captain, 83

cosmeceuticals, 17

cosmetic care remedies

    Anti-Acne "Spot Not" Mask, 162

    Antifungal Nail Treatment, 186

    Anti-Stretch Mark Belly Rub,
        191

    Basic Bath Salts, 171

    Basic Body Butter, 169

    Basic Lip Balm, 165

    Citrus-Flower Body Butter, 170

    Citrus Serum for Combination
        Skin, 176

    Easy Whipped Moisturizer, 175

    Frankincense and Common
        Sense Serum, 164

    Geranium Lip Scrub, 167

    Green Tea Toner, 174

Healing Heels Salve, 185

Hot Oil Treatment for Brittle Hair, 177

Lavender-Rosehip Face Oil, 188

Lavender-Rosemary Hair Thickening Treatment, 180

Lemon-Lavender Lip Balm, 166

Neroli Replenishing Hand Cream, 182

Nourishing Cuticle Lotion, 187

Nourishing Nighttime Lotion, 163

Orange-Patchouli Gardening Soap, 184

Peppermint Massage Gel, 183

Post-Pregnancy Stretch Mark Slather, 190

Rosacea Treatment for Mature Skin, 189

Rosemary and Cedarwood Dandruff Shampoo, 178

Sandalwood Serum, 168

Scalp-Stimulating Conditioner, 181

Spicy Lime Salt Scrub, 173

Tea Tree-Orange Dandruff Treatment, 179

Winter Warming Coffee Body Scrub, 172

cosmetic clay ingredients, 239–240

cosmetic plants, 17

cost-effectiveness, 26

cough drops, 110

coughs, 109–110

cradle cap, 113–114

cranberry juice, 154

Crusaders, 15

curse of the Celts, 188

curses, 128

cuts, 115–116

cypress essential oil, 19

D

dandruff, 178–179

dementia, 14

deodorant, 103

depression, 117–119

    aromatherapy, 15

desensitized sense of smell, 21, 27

diabetes, 96, 159

diaper rash, 54, 120–121

Diaz, Cameron, 188

digestive problems, 122–123

Dior, 74, 75

Diptych, 232

distillation, 16

dogs

    Baby-Safe Salve, 126

    calming spray, 219

    ticks, 218

drain cleaner, 208

dry skin, 168–170, 172–173, 175

Durant, Will, 15

dust mites, 215

E

ear infections, 124–125

earthy essential oils, 30

eau de cologne, 226–227

eau de parfum, 221–223

eau de toilette, 221, 224–225

eczema, 126–127

Eddie Bauer, 67

Egyptians, 9, 51, 54, 68, 76, 229

    masceration, 18

    mummification process, 15

emmenagogues, 22

emollient, 232

Encre Noire, 84

enfleurage, 18

Epsom salts, 119

erectile dysfunction, 128–129

essential equipment, 35–37

essential oil-infused recipes, 17

essential oils, 14

    abortifacient, 22

    allergies, 22

    ancient history and, 9

    to avoid, 24

    beeswax and, 146

best ways to apply, 34

blending, 24–26

brand reputation, 31

brands, 236–237

buying too many at once, 46

candle makers, 9

certified, 31

children and, 24

citrus essential oils, 30

CO_2 extraction, 18

cruelty-free, 27

defining, 16

desensitized sense of smell, 21, 27

diluting, 19–20

earthy essential oils, 30

emmenagogues, 22

enfleurage, 18

expression, 18

eyes and, 21

fat-soluble compounds, 16

flammability, 21

floral essential oils, 30

frequency of use, 21, 27

half-strength recipes, 24

health care uses, 19–20

herbaceous essential oils, 30

holistic approach to health, 14

home products, 34

improperly storing, 46

ingestion, 20, 34

inhalation, 19, 34

maceration, 18

marketing claims, 31

massage therapists, 9

measurement dilutions and conversions, 45

medications and, 21

medicinal essential oils, 30

metabolizing, 21, 27

minty essential oils, 30

oriental essential oils, 30

overusing, 21

patch test, 20–21

photosensitization, 16, 22
pregnancy, 22
prices, 30–31, 50
producing, 18–19
purity, 30
quick reference guide, 234–235
relationships with, 23
safety, 20–22, 24
scent, 30
senior citizens and, 24
sensitization, 16, 21
shelf life, 30
shopping for, 30–31
solvent extraction, 19
spicy essential oils, 30
steam distillation, 18
strength, 16
synergy, 20
therapeutic uses, 21
topical application, 19–20, 34
using too much, 45–46
woody essential oils, 30
eucalyptus essential oil, 19, 40, 44
Eudora, 53
evaporative diffusers, 34
Everglades, 73
exfoliation, 112, 171–173
expression, 18
eyes and essential oils, 21

F

face care
    combination skin, 176
    dry skin, 175
    oily skin, 174
facials, 14
facial serums, 176
febrefuge, 232
fever blisters, 102
fig leaf essential oil, 24
Fille en Aiguilles, 80
fir essential oil, 19
First Nation, 17
flammability, 21

Fleur Classique Parfum, 223
Fleur Poivrée, 53
floral essential oils, 30
floral waters. *See* hydrosols
Florida Water, 17
flour, 115
flower waters. *See* hydrosols
flu, 130–131
foaming soap dispenser, 98
food coloring, 171
foot odor, 93–95
fragrance notes, 24–26
fragrance oils, 16
fragrances, 24
French lavender (*Lavandula stoechas*), 22
fungus, 94

G

garages and mold, 210
garden sprays, 216–217
garlic oil, 124
garlic oil-enriched eye salve, 17
gas, 122
geranium essential oil, 20, 218
German chamomile essential oil, 56
gifts, 27
    customized bath salts, 119
Givenchy, 85
glass cleaner, 209
glycerin, 172
grapefruit essential oil, 20
grapeseed oil, 33
Greeks, 15, 55, 68, 76, 229
Guerlain, 74
Guerlain, Pierre-François Pascal, 227

H

hair care
    brittle hair, 177
    dandruff, 178, 179
    hair loss, 181
    hair thickening, 180

half-strength recipes for essential oils, 24
hand and foot care, 182–185
handmade candles, 27
hand washing, 131
Harris, Lea, 32
hazelnut oil, 34
headaches, 132–133
health and healing remedies, 87–88
    Abscess Relieving Compress, 137
    Antibacterial Soap with Rosemary and Thyme, 98
    Antifungal Lotion for Ringworm, 139
    Antiseptic Spray, 136
    Anti-Sting Bee Sting Paste, 100
    Baby Bum Lotion, 121
    Baby-Safe Salve, 126
    Basic Burn Gel, 107
    Basic Mouthwash, 96
    Basic Warming Oil, 91
    Chamomile-Calendula Diaper Cream, 120
    Chamomile Sunburn Gel, 151
    Clove Anti-Itch Cream, 127
    Comfrey Bruise Healing Oil, 105
    Cooling Sunburn Spritz, 152
    De-Stress Bath Salts, 119
    Diffuser Blends That Help SAD, 147
    Digestion Bath, 112
    The Easiest Mosquito Bite Remedy Ever, 99
    Essential Cradle Cap Oil Blend, 113
    Eucalyptus-Mint Rub, 109
    Eucalyptus-Sandalwood Sinus Relief, 149
    Five Flower Balm, 118
    Four-Oil Hemorrhoid Blend, 134
    Frankincense Flu Rub, 130
    Freeze-Out Fever Blister Ointment, 102
    Gas Relief Rub, 122
    Gentle Lavender Oil Blend, 114

Geranium-Calendula Blister Gel, 101

Ginger Lotion, 143

Happiness Is a Warm Bath, 117

Herbal Indigestion Massage, 123

High Performance Blend Massage Oil, 128

Hormone Help Bath, 141

Lavender-Eucalyptus Diffuser Blend, 132

Lavender-Tea Tree Lice Treatment, 138

Massage Lotion for Babies, 90

The Medicinal Compress, 155

Minty Mineralizing Toothpaste, 97

Mood Elevating Spritz, 148

Myrrh Mouthwash for Toothache, 153

No Sweat Mist, 140

Numbing Sunburn Spray, 108

Palmarosa PMS Massage Oil, 145

Peppermint-Lemon Headache Oil, 133

Pickle Your Toes Foot Bath, 94

PMS Blend Votive Candle, 146

Rejuvenating Juniper Bath Soak, 144

Rosemary-Lavender Salve for Bruises, 106

Rosemary-Lemon-Eucalyptus Rub, 110

Sanitizing Hand Gel, 131

Sinus-Soothing Diffuser Blend, 150

Smothering the Fire Oil, 92

Soothing Hemorrhoid Treatment, 135

Spearmint Anti-Nausea Drops, 142

Spice-It-Up Bath Blend, 129

Stinky Feet Soak, 95

Swimmer's Ear Relief, 125

Take a Deep Breath Calming Diffusion Oil, 89

The Tamanu-Tea Tree Bath, 154

Tea Tree and Juniper Body Wash, 104

Tea Tree and Lavender Foot Powder, 93

Tea Tree Gel, 116

Tea Tree Internal Salve, 158

Tea Tree & Lemon Deodorant, 103

Tea Tree Oil Treatment, 115, 124

Twisted Sister Varicose Vein Body Butter, 156

Unclench Massage Blend, 111

Varicose Vein Massage Oil Blends, 157

Yogurt and Tea Tree Remedy, 159

health care uses for essential oils, 19–20

heartburn, 122–123

heat diffusers, 34

helichrysum essential oil, 105

Helichrysum (*Helichrysum italicum*), 191

hemorrhoids, 134–135

herbaceous essential oils, 30

Herb Society of America, 76

herpes, 102

hexane, 19

Hildegard of Bingen, 74

Hindi temples, 54

Hippocrates, 76, 100

Hirsch, Alan, 129

Hittites, 76

holistic approach to health, 14

home
  essential oils, 34
  reducing toxic chemicals, 26

home remedies
  After-Workout Antifungal Spray, 199
  Bathtub Ring Banisher, 198
  Calming Spray for Dogs, 219
  Carpet Spot Remover for Synthetic Fibers, 202
  Citronella-Peppermint Mosquito Repellent, 211

Citrus Cheer Diffuser Blend, 194

Citrus Drain Flush, 208

Citrus-Vinegar Disinfectant Spray, 201

DIY Glass Cleaner, 209

DIY Laundry Stain Remover, 205

Dust Mite Deterrent, 215

Fizzy Tea Tree Toilet Cleaner, 200

Homemade Dryer Sheets, 204

Kitchen Grease-Busting Cleaner, 197

Linen Water, 207

Natural Spot Remover for Natural Fiber Carpets, 203

Nix Ticks Blend for Dogs, 218

Nontoxic Weed Killer, 216

Old-Fashioned Laundry Detergent, 206

Pepper Spray for Plant Pests, 217

Roach Spray, 213

Roll-On Geranium Bug Repellent, 212

Simple Citrus Air Freshener, 195

Simple Spider Spray, 214

Tea Tree Anti-Mold Spray, 210

Thieves' Oil All-Purpose Cleaner, 196

Hoodoo folk magic, 81

hormone imbalance, 141

horseradish essential oil, 24

hot flashes, 140

Hoyt's Cologne, 17

human touch, 90

humectant, 232

Hungary Water, 17, 227

hydrosols, 16, 18

I

impacted wisdom teeth, 153

India, 53, 69, 82

Indian rose, 77

indigestion, 123

indolic, 232

infantile seborrheic dermatitis, 113

infants. *See* babies

infections, 136–137

ingestion, 20, 34

ingredients

    bath salts, 237

    beauty butters, 238

    bottles, containers, & jars, 238

    candles, 239

    cosmetic clay, 239–240

    soap making, 240

inhalation, 19, 34

insect repellent, 211–215

insoluble, 233

J

J'ai Osé Aqua, 67

Jasmin 17, 77

jasmine essential oil, 31

jojoba oil, 16, 19, 33

Joy, 232

juniper essential oil, 144

K

Kahun Gynaecological Papyrus, 140

Kananga Water, 17

Karan, Donna, 229

khus oil, 84

kidney disease, 96

kitchen cleaner, 197

L

Lalique, 84

Laroche, Guy, 67

laundry, 204–207

Lavandula angustifolia, 22

lavender essential oil, 17, 20, 26, 40

    Five Thieves' Disinfectant Spray, 44

    Lavender Moisturizing Hand Cream, 43

lavender (*Lavandula augustifolia*) essential oil, 90

leechbooks, 17

Le Labo, 77

lemon balm essential oil (Melissa oil), 30

lemon essential oil, 20, 40

    Five Thieves' Disinfectant Spray, 44

    Lemon-Peppermint Lip Balm, 42

lemongrass essential oil, 20

lice, 138–139

licorice root, 122

limbic system, 19

Lime, 71

Lime Rickey, 71

limey, 71

lower esophageal sphinter (LES), 123

Lutens, Sergei, 78, 80

M

macadamia nut oil, 35

maceration, 18

Magi, 9

Malaysia, 85

Mao Zedong, 96

Mark Antony, 164

marketing claims, 31

massage oils, 129

massages, 14

massage therapists, 9

measurement conversions, 231

medications and essential oils, 21

medicinal essential oils, 30

medicinal plants, 17

medicine and orange essential oil, 89

medieval era, 9

Melissa oil. *See* lemon balm

Mencken, H.L., 198

menopause, 140–141

methylene chloride, 19

Micozzi, Marc, 14

microfiber towels, 209

Middleton, Catherine, 142

migraines, 132

Miller, Bryan, 80

Miller, Light, 80

mint essential oil, 19

minty essential oils, 30

Miss Dior Cherie L'Eau, 75

moisturizers, 168–170

mold, 210

morning sickness, 142–143

mosquito bites, 99

mosquito repellent, 211

mother-infant bond, 90

moth repellents, 55

MRSA, 17, 83

Mugler, Thierry, 78

multipurpose products, 26

muscle aches, 143

mustard essential oil, 24

N

nail care, 186–187

nail fungus, 186

nard. *See* spikenard

National Cancer Institute, 19

Native Americans, 17

nausea, 143

neat, 233

nebulizers, 34

"The Neglected Anniversary," 198

New Testament, 9

No. 5, 232

O

oatmeal, 151

O'Donnell, Rosie, 188

oily skin, 174

Old Spice Lime, 71

Olene, 232

olfactory bulb, 19

Ombre D'Or, 85

orange essential oil, 17, 31, 89

oriental essential oils, 30

osteoarthritis, 91

outhouses, 200

oven temperatures, 231

overeating, 123

over-the-counter medicines
  alternatives, 26

P

palmarosa essential oil, 20
paperbark tree, 73
Parfums 06130, 229
Patchouli, 78
patchouli essential oil, 25
patch test, 20–21
Patou, Jean, 232
pennyroyal essential oil, 24
peppermint essential oil, 20, 31, 40
  Lemon-Peppermint Lip Balm, 42
perfume oils. *See* fragrance oils
perfume recipes, 222
  Fleur Classique Parfum, 223
  Garden in the Woods Eau De
    Toilette, 224
  Healing Aftershave Splash, 229
  Hungary Water, 227
  Lavender-Lemon Eau De
    Toilette, 225
  A Night in Marrakesh Solid
    Perfume, 222
  Unisex Citrus & Spice Splash,
    228
  Winter Spice Cologne, 226
perfumes, 15
  alcohol-based, 17
  fixing citrus scents, 74
  scents, 25
perfume tree, 85
Persians, 15
pets, 218–219
Phaedon, 84
Philippines, 85
photosensitization, 16, 22
phototoxic, 233
piles, 134
Pliny, 74
Popy Moreni, 53
porous materials for mixing,
    measuring, and pouring, 46
post-pregnancy, 190

pot marigold. *See* calendula
    essential oil
pregnancy and essential oils, 22
premenstrual syndrome (PMS),
    145–146
prep equipment, 35
product quality, 27
Public Enemy, 66
purity, 30

R

ragweed allergies, 22, 56
rashes, 126–127
recipes, essential oil-infused, 17
repelling insects, 20
Revlon, 77
ringworm, 138–139
Roman chamomile essential
    oil, 20, 56
Romans, 9, 15, 51, 55, 68, 79, 229
rosacea, 188–189
rose essential oil, 17, 31
rose geranium, 77
rosehip seed oils, 33
rosemary essential oil, 20
rose otto. *See* attar of roses, 17
roses, 17
rosewater (*golab*), 15
Ruhl Bee Supply website, 239

S

sandalwood essential oil, 20
sassafras essential oil, 24
savin essential oil, 24
scars, 191
scents
  essential oils, 30
  perfumes, 25
  signature scent, 27
Seasonal Affective Disorder
    (SAD), 147–148
senior citizens
  essential oils, 24
  Smothering the Fire Oil, 92
sensitization, 16, 19–21, 27, 233

Shabistari, Mahmud, 15
shaker tops, 93
Shakespeare, 81
shea butter, 118, 169
Shirley Temple, 71
shopping for aromatherapy
    projects, 29–27
  carrier oils, 31, 33–35
  core ingredients, 30–35
  essential equipment, 35–37
  essential oils, 30–31
  odds and ends, 37
  prep equipment, 35
  storage equipment, 36–37
  where to buy items for, 37
Shutes, Jade, 23, 31
signature scent, 27
sinus pain, 149–150
skin rejuvenation, 164
sleep-inducing essential oils, 20
Smell and Taste Treatment and
    Research Foundation, 129
Smith Brothers, 110
snakeroot essential oil, 24
soap making ingredients, 240
sodium carbonate, 206
solvent extraction, 19
spa industry, 14
Spanish lavender, 22
spicy essential oils, 30
spiders, 214
spike lavender (*Lavandula
    latifolia*), 22
spikenard, 15
splashes, 221, 228–229
spruce essential oil, 19
Sri Lanka, 70
steam distillation, 15, 18
stewing herbs, 202
stings, 98–99
storage equipment, 36–37
stress, 133
  foot odor, 95
  management, 20

stretch marks, 190–191
Sufi metaphysics, 15
summer depression, 147
sunburn, 108, 151–152
sweet almond oil, 19, 33
sweet cicely, 72
swimmer's ear, 125
swollen joints, 92
synergy, 20

T

Talmud, 72
tea tree (black) essential oil
    (*Melaleuca bracteata*), 24
tea tree essential oil, 24, 31, 40, 44
Theophrastus of Athens, 15
thermogenic, 233
thieves' oil, 17, 26
Thieves' Oil All-Purpose
    Cleaner, 196
thuja essential oil, 24
thyme essential oil, 20
toenail fungus, 186
toilet cleaner, 200, 201
toilet water, 17
toothache, 153

toothpaste, 97
topical application, 34
toxic chemicals, 26
Tree of Life (*arborvitae*), 55
Turkish rose, 77

U

ultrasonic/humidifying
    diffusers, 34
undiluted oils, 45
urinary tract infection
    (UTI), 154–155

V

varicose veins, 156–157
Venus, 17
vermifuge, 233
vetiver, 84
Vetiver Sport, 74
Vicks VapoRub, 109
Vietnam, 53
Villoresi, Lorenzo, 78
Virgin Mary, 17
volume equivalents (dry), 231
volume equivalents (liquid), 231

W

Walmart, 209
walnut oil, 35
washing soda, 206
weed killer, 216
weight equivalents, 231
Whole Foods, 169
Wiccan rituals, 78
wicks, 239
woody essential oils, 30
wormwood essential oil, 24

X

xylitol, 97

Y

yeast infection, 158–159
Ylang Austral, 85
ylang ylang essential oil, 17, 25

Z

Zara, 84
Zellweger, Renée, 188
Zhisui, Li, 96

IMAGE CREDITS

PHOTOGRAPHY

Cover: © barol16; © Shannon Douglas (back cover); © Tom Bringham (illustrations on flaps and throughout)

Alamy: © Radius Images: 160

Dreamstime: © Wasanajai: 78

© Shannon Douglas: 3, 11, 28, 47, 230

iStock: © botamochi: 23; © Chris Gramly: 192

Shutterstock: © Abyzova Elena: 55; © Africa Studio, 66; © alybaba: 73; © Antonova Anna: 12; © B and E Dudzinscy: 51; © Bildagentur Zoonar GmbH: 59; © blueeyes: 68; © Calvste: 57; © Celig: throughout (wood surface); © chanwangrong: 75;

© Chayapak Maspan: 77; © DC_Aperture: 76; © efirm: 80; © Everything: 53; © forest71: 52; © Gayvoronskaya_Yana: 48; © grafvision: 65; © Hitdelight: 50; © hjochen: 63; © janaph: 62; © Juta: 79; © kajornyot wildlife photography: 85; © Kao-len: 70; © Karves: 60; © Malchus Kern: 72; © Thanthima Lima: 84; © long8614: 61; © longtail-dog: 67; © Verena Matthew: 64; © Melpomene: 38; © Pawel Michalowski: 71; © Claus Mikosch: 81; © picturepartners: 83; © pryzmat: 54; © PSD photography: 57; © Luisa Puccini: 86; © R_Szatkowski: 74; © sakschaistockphoto: 58; © Scorpp: 56; © Oksana Shufrych: 220; © Igor Sirbu: 41; © Olaf Speier: 69; © ZIGROUP-CREATIONS: 82

Thinkstock: © barol16: 6; © natashamam: 25

ILLUSTRATIONS

© Tom Bingham